LIVING WITH PARKINSON'S DISEASE

BRIDGET McCALL worked for 17 years for the Parkinson's Disease Society (PDS) and developed close links with many people with Parkinson's and their families. She has written widely on Parkinson's and has produced a wide variety of information resources, electronic and audio-visual.

D1077523

Overcoming Common Problems Series

Selected titles

A full list of titles is available from Sheldon Press,
36 Causton Street, London SW1P 4ST and on our website at
www.sheldonpress.co.uk

Overcoming Common Problems

Living With Parkinson's Disease

Bridget McCall

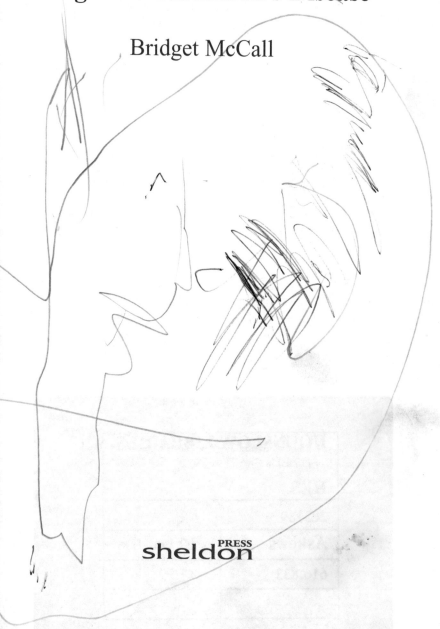

sheldon**PRESS**

First published in Great Britain in 2006

Sheldon Press
36 Causton Street
London SW1P 4ST

The author and publisher have made every effort to ensure that the external
website addresses included in this book are correct and up to date at the time of
going to press. The author and publisher are not responsible for the content,
quality or continuing accessibility of sites.

British Library Cataloguing-in-Publication Data
A catalogue record for this book is available from the British Library

ISBN-13: 978–0–85969–957–0
ISBN-10: 0–85969–957–9

1 3 5 7 9 10 8 6 4 2

Typeset by Avocet Typeset, Chilton, Aylesbury, Bucks
Printed in Great Britain by Ashford Colour Press

Contents

Acknowledgements

I would particularly like to thank all the people with Parkinson's, their partners and family members who contributed personal experiences to this book. As some wanted to appear under a pseudonym I have not listed them by name. I am extremely grateful to them all for the time they gave me and their willingness to share their stories with me and the readers of this book. Also the many people with Parkinson's, carers and health and social care professionals that I met and worked with during my employment at the Parkinson's Disease Society (PDS), who taught me so much about Parkinson's.

I would also like to acknowledge the many published resources on Parkinson's disease, listed in Further reading, which I have used as references while writing this book and in particular the many publications produced by the Parkinson's Disease Society.

I would also like to thank the following people who provided information, helped me set up interviews, commented on drafts or simply gave me much needed moral support while I was writing this book: Rena Brewin, Paulo Mata and the staff of the Islington Princess Royal Trust Carers Centre, Anne Bridge, Dr David Burn, John Bucknall, Frances Carroll, Marilyn Caven, Barbara Cormie, Colin Cosgrove, Jane Daniels, Wendy Darch, Dr Duncan Forsyth, Pat Good, Professor Marwan Hariz, Rosie Hayward, Julie Henbury, Linda and Brian Hill, Fiona Marshall, Chris McCall, Joe and Rosemary McCall, Dr Paul Morrish, Sue Peckitt, Diana Pert, Ian Prest, Jenny, Pam and Neil Russell, Val Southwell, Abi Vernon, Sheila Windsor and Fiona, Thomas and Michael Youngman.

Introduction

If you are reading this book, the chances are that you or someone close to you has Parkinson's disease. You are probably looking for information to help you understand more about Parkinson's and how best to cope with it. I hope this book will answer the questions you have about the nature of Parkinson's, its treatment and the support available.

The contents are based on my many years' experience of working with people with Parkinson's, their relatives, and the health and social care professionals who provide support. This includes my previous work at the Parkinson's Disease Society of the United Kingdom, where I spent over 17 years answering questions and producing information about Parkinson's and related subjects. In my current role as a freelance writer and editor, my work continues to include many Parkinson's projects – including this book!

Although factual information is vitally important, and the book includes plenty of this, experience has taught me that the real experts are the people who live with Parkinson's every day. I hope the stories and insights from the people I have interviewed for this book will inspire you. I hope they demonstrate that, although living with Parkinson's may not always be easy and sometimes adjustments have to be made to accommodate Parkinson's, it is still possible to have a good quality of life.

The following points were stressed by the people I interviewed:

- Parkinson's is a complicated condition that affects everyone differently – in terms of symptoms, response to medication and the way it progresses. Don't assume that you will experience everything that is mentioned in this book.
- There is no right or wrong way to cope with Parkinson's – you have to find out what works best for you.
- Never give up hope. Help is available. There have been many scientific and medical advances in the understanding and treatment of Parkinson's in recent years, including several new drugs and a renewed interest in surgical techniques. Many more are on the horizon.

If you want more information on any of the subjects discussed in this book, details of resources and organizations that can help you further are given in Useful addresses.

1

What is Parkinson's disease?

Parkinson's is known to have existed since ancient times – Galen, the second-century Greek–Roman physician, described at least two types of tremor. It first became a recognized medical condition in 1817 with the publication of Dr James Parkinson's famous description of the disease, *An Essay on the Shaking Palsy*. Dr Parkinson (1755–1824) was a pioneering London doctor who wrote widely on medical, scientific and political issues of his day. His essay on Parkinson's was based on observations he had made of six cases in his own practice in Hoxton in east London. His descriptions are incomplete because he was able to examine only one of these six people, but his account is considered remarkable, even by today's sophisticated medical standards, for its accuracy and clear expression.

James Parkinson hoped that his essay would encourage others to study the condition – and so it proved. Several nineteenth-century doctors, including the famous French neurologist Jean-Martin Charcot, studied the condition. In the twentieth century, many further advances were made, especially in the last 20–30 years. In the twenty-first century, this trend is continuing. The 250th anniversary of Dr Parkinson's birth occurred on 11 April 2005. If he were alive today, he would be astonished and delighted at the progress that has been made in the understanding and treatment of the condition that bears his name.

What is Parkinson's?

Parkinson's disease is a progressive, neurological condition that has three main symptoms:

- tremor;
- rigidity; and
- slowness of movement (bradykinesia).

Parkinson's generally begins slowly, often in an arm or a leg on one side of the body, and people often have vague symptoms for at least a year, or longer, before the symptoms start to interfere with everyday activities or become noticeable enough to prompt the person to seek medical advice. Although the symptoms will remain predominantly one-sided in some people, in many cases they eventually develop on both sides of the body.

Tremor is the symptom that people instantly identify with Parkinson's. Yet up to 30 per cent of people with Parkinson's don't experience this symptom. Also, there are several distinct types of tremor, which have different causes. People with Parkinson's have a 'resting tremor' – it tends to occur when the affected part of the body is at rest, and lessens when it is in use.

As a result of the symptoms of rigidity and slowness of movement, people with Parkinson's find that their movements feel stiff, become unco-ordinated and more difficult to initiate, and take longer to perform. Fine movements of the fingers are often the first to be affected, and problems with handwriting may result, for example. There may also be difficulty turning around, getting out of a chair or turning over in bed. Walking, posture and balance can also be affected. Many people experience difficulties with movements that are involved in communication, such as speech, facial expression and body language. Tiredness and depression are also common features (see Chapter 3).

If you are newly diagnosed with Parkinson's, it can be very frightening to read a list of symptoms like this. Remember that Parkinson's is a very individual condition that affects each person differently with regard to symptoms, the nature and speed of their development, and the response to treatment. You may never have some of the symptoms and experiences described in this book.

Many people ask if Parkinson's is a fatal illness. With today's treatments, in most cases life expectancy is roughly the same as it is for people in general. Sometimes Parkinson's may weaken the health of someone who has had the condition for many years and be a contributory factor to other illnesses that do cause death.

Parkinsonism

The main symptoms of Parkinson's (tremor, rigidity and bradykinesia) are also key features of a group of conditions collectively known as parkinsonism.

The most common type of parkinsonism is idiopathic Parkinson's disease (usually described as Parkinson's disease), which about 85 per cent of people diagnosed with parkinsonism have. Idiopathic means 'of unknown cause', which is misleading because several other types of parkinsonism also have unknown causes.

The remaining 15 per cent generally have other, rarer forms of parkinsonism. These include essential tremor, corticobasal degeneration, multiple system atrophy, progressive supranuclear palsy, drug-induced parkinsonism, vascular parkinsonism and dementia with Lewy bodies.

Doctors sometimes divide parkinsonism conditions into two classes:

- akinetic–rigid syndromes, which are characterized by stiffness and lack of movement – these syndromes include corticobasal degeneration, progressive supranuclear palsy and multiple system atrophy; and
- hyperkinetic syndromes, which are associated with excessive movement, such as essential tremor.[1]

Distinguishing between these different forms of parkinsonism can sometimes be difficult because, with the exception of essential tremor, there are no medical tests that can establish whether a person has Parkinson's or one of the other forms of parkinsonism (see Chapter 4).

Other types of parkinsonism

Corticobasal degeneration

Corticobasal degeneration (CBD) is a rare form of parkinsonism that has some similarities with progressive supranuclear palsy (see below). It can present in several different ways and, in addition to causing parkinsonism symptoms, it can affect mental processes such as memory, vision perception, speech, organizational skills, personality and behaviour. Corticobasal degeneration tends to be asymmetrical (on one side). A particular feature is the 'alien limb' phenomenon, where the person's limb seems to move without control, as if it had a mind of its own.[2] Care focuses on management to ensure quality of life.

Further information is available from either the Pick's Disease Support Group or the PSP (Europe) Association.

Dementia with Lewy bodies[3]

Dementia with Lewy bodies (DLB) is a dementia that shares characteristics with both Alzheimer's and Parkinson's. It gets its name from the microscopic deposits called Lewy bodies that are found after death in certain parts of the brains of people with the condition. The presence of these Lewy bodies in the brain disrupts the brain's normal functioning. Lewy bodies are also found in idiopathic Parkinson's disease but their extent and pattern of distribution in the two conditions is quite different. In addition to the symptoms of dementia, about 75 per cent of people with dementia with Lewy bodies also develop parkinsonism symptoms. Features that are particularly characteristic of dementia with Lewy bodies include fainting; falling; detailed and convincing visual hallucinations (often of people or animals); and falling asleep very easily by day but having restless, disturbed nights with confusion, nightmares and hallucinations. People with this condition find that their abilities often fluctuate daily or even hourly.

While there is no cure for dementia with Lewy bodies, the drugs for Parkinson's may be used to treat the parkinsonism symptoms, although the response is usually less good than it is in people with Parkinson's. Research suggests that the cholinesterase inhibitor drugs used to treat Alzheimer's disease, such as donepezil hydrochloride (*Aricept*), rivastigmine (*Exelon*) and galantamine (*Reminyl*) may be useful for treating dementia with Lewy bodies, although they are not yet licensed for this use. However, any improvement is likely to be modest.

Further information and support for people who have dementia with Lewy bodies and their families can be obtained from the Alzheimer's Society, Alzheimer Scotland – Action on Dementia or the Pick's Disease Support Group.

Drug-induced parkinsonism[4]

About 7 per cent of people with parkinsonism develop it after taking certain medications, and some who already have parkinsonism find that their symptoms worsen if they are treated with these medications. The drugs in question are those that block the action of dopamine (the neurotransmitter in the brain that is in short supply in the brains of people with Parkinson's disease). Drugs of particular note are the antipsychotic or neuroleptic drugs used to treat schizophrenia and other psychotic problems;

prochlorperazine (*Stemetil*) used to treat dizziness and nausea; and metoclopromide (*Maxolon*) used to treat nausea and indigestion. There are however several others as well (see Chapter 6).

Treatment is usually to stop the offending drug or reduce the dose, or to change to another drug. Sometimes, for medical reasons, none of these may be possible, in which case the doctor, in consultation with the patient, will need to weigh up the benefits of the drug against the side-effects of parkinsonism.

If you think you might have drug-induced parkinsonism, you should discuss this with your doctor. Don't stop any medication you have been prescribed before you have done this as some drugs have to be withdrawn slowly to avoid any problems that can occur as a result of stopping them suddenly.

Theoretically, illegal drugs such as cocaine, ecstasy and heroin can also be causes of drug-induced parkinsonism, although research in this area is limited. In the late 1970s and early 1980s some drug addicts in the USA rapidly developed parkinsonism symptoms when they took a designer drug that was synthesized to produce similar effects to heroin. This synthesized drug was found to contain a substance called MPTP (1-methyl-4-phenyl-1,2,3,6-tetrahydropyridine), which the body converted into a specific toxin called MPP+. This toxin caused the death of the dopamine-producing neurones (nerve cells) in the substantia nigra.[5] (See also page 11.)

Essential tremor[6]

Essential tremor is a common neurological condition whereby people may experience rhythmic trembling of the hands, head, legs, trunk or voice. This tremor is different from the Parkinson's resting tremor – it is an action tremor that is more obvious when the affected part of the body is in use or when the arms are outstretched.

Essential tremor, unlike Parkinson's, often runs in families. It affects men and women equally and it affects people of any age. Essential tremor, particularly in older people, can be difficult to differentiate from Parkinson's, and misdiagnosis is common. However, diagnosis is becoming easier because of the development of a radiopharmaceutical agent, DaTSCAN, which doctors can use with neuroimaging to differentiate essential tremor from other causes of parkinsonism. DaTSCAN cannot, however, diagnose idiopathic Parkinson's or distinguish it from other forms of parkinsonism.

Essential tremor is progressive and people with it may find that some of their functional abilities are affected, causing them to have problems with such activities as handwriting, holding things in the hands and fine manipulation.

Although there is no cure, treatment is available. Drugs may be prescribed to control the tremor, including anticonvulsants, beta-blockers and benzodiazepines, or a combination of a beta-blocker and an anticonvulsant. Small amounts of alcohol may suppress the symptoms in some people. In severe cases, surgery or botulinum toxin injections may also be considered.

For more information contact the National Tremor Foundation.

Multiple system atrophy[7]

Multiple system atrophy (MSA) is a progressive neurological condition of unknown cause, with three groups of symptoms:

- parkinsonism;
- cerebellar symptoms, including difficulties in co-ordinating movement and balance; and
- autonomic difficulties (that is, problems with automatic body functions such as bladder control, sweating, and blood pressure; for men, the first sign is often erectile dysfunction; low blood pressure, resulting in feelings of dizziness or fainting, can also be a problem.

Multiple system atrophy progresses more quickly than Parkinson's.

Treatment is similar to that used for Parkinson's, although response to the Parkinson's drugs is generally less good.

For more information contact the Sarah Matheson Trust for Multiple System Atrophy.

Post-encephalitic parkinsonism

Between 1916 and 1926 there was a worldwide epidemic of a viral infection called encephalitis lethargica. Some people who had this infection subsequently developed a rare, severe form of parkinsonism known as post-encephalitic parkinsonism. In his famous book, *Awakenings*, later made into a film starring Robin Williams and Robert de Niro, the neurologist Dr Oliver Sacks documented his work in New York with patients with post-encephalitic parkinsonism and his attempts in the late 1960s to treat them with levodopa, then an experimental drug. Today there are few people still alive who were affected by the encephalitis lethargica epidemic, and new cases are rare.[8]

Progressive supranuclear palsy[9]

Progressive supranuclear palsy (PSP) is the commonest of the akinetic–rigid syndromes. As well as the rigidity and bradykinesia associated with Parkinson's, people with this condition experience difficulties in moving the eyes – for example, they may find it difficult or impossible to look down voluntarily. Balance problems, early falls, and problems with speech and swallowing are also characteristic of progressive supranuclear palsy. The symptoms tend to occur on both sides of the body at once and progression is usually more rapid that it is for idiopathic Parkinson's disease.

Treatment is similar to that for Parkinson's, although response to the Parkinson's drugs is generally less good.

For more information contact the PSP (Europe) Association.

Vascular (or arteriosclerotic) parkinsonism[10]

Strokes, which affect more than 130,000 people in England and Wales each year, do not cause Parkinson's, but several small strokes in a part of the brain called the corpus striatum may result in parkinsonism symptoms, such as rigidity and slowness; a tendency to walk with short, shuffling steps; and some difficulty speaking clearly. The corpus striatum is linked to the substantia nigra, the part of the brain affected in Parkinson's (see Chapter 2).

Stroke symptoms appear suddenly and do not progress, whereas Parkinson's symptoms appear slowly and do progress. With a stroke, symptoms may go away, though they don't always, whereas in Parkinson's they don't. However, with minor strokes, the person may not even be aware of the event, in which case symptoms may progress gradually and resemble the progression of idiopathic Parkinson's disease.

The main aim of treatment is to try and lower the chance of further strokes by trying to control risk factors – such as giving up smoking; eating a low-fat, low-salt diet; and taking regular exercise. Treatment of the parkinsonism symptoms is difficult because vascular parkinsonism does not generally respond well to Parkinson's medication and elderly people may be more prone to develop side-effects.

For more information on strokes, contact the Stroke Association. (See also Chapter 13.)

2

Who gets Parkinson's disease and why?

In the UK about 100,000 people have Parkinson's and about 10,000 people are newly diagnosed with it each year.[11] It is more common in people aged 60 and over, with the prevalence increasing with age – Parkinson's affects about one in 100 people over the age of 65 and one in 50 people over the age of 80.[12] However, younger people can also have Parkinson's – one in 20 people diagnosed with it are under the age 40.[13]

Parkinson's affects people in all parts of the world. Men and women are affected more or less equally, although some studies suggest that the condition is more common in men.

Why Parkinson's happens

Parkinson's is a disorder of the brain, an enormously complicated organ that monitors and co-ordinates both our unconscious (autonomic or automatic) and our voluntary actions. It also houses our consciousness, used for thinking, learning and creativity.

Parkinson's occurs because the brain stops producing enough dopamine, a neurotransmitter involved in the control of voluntary movements. Dopamine is produced in the substantia nigra (which simply means 'black substance'), a black, pigmented section of the basal ganglia, the part of the brain that co-ordinates muscle and body movements. Dopamine works as a chemical messenger sending signals to other parts of the brain. It plays an important role in helping to control movement and balance and in maintaining proper functioning of the central nervous system.

In normal circumstances the cells in the substantia nigra generate most of the dopamine in the body. In Parkinson's, these dopamine-producing cells begin to degenerate, gradually and progressively over a number of years. Symptoms become obvious only as the disease progresses, and they may start to appear when about 70–80 per cent of the dopamine cells have been lost.

The main processes of the brain that are affected by this loss of dopamine are those involving voluntary movements rather than autonomic functions or consciousness, which explains the three main symptoms of tremor, rigidity and slowness of movement.

One of the most frustrating aspects of Parkinson's is that, although we know that it results from the loss of dopamine in the brain, we don't know why this happens. Areas of interest to researchers include ageing, genetics, environmental factors and viruses. Some researchers have suggested that Parkinson's may turn out to be more than one condition, having several causes.

Ageing

Ageing can clearly play some role in the development of Parkinson's and can affect and interact with Parkinson's symptoms. However, ageing by itself can't explain Parkinson's because younger people can develop it and the type of dopamine loss seen in Parkinson's disease differs from that seen in normal ageing.[14] Some studies have also suggested that people who are very elderly (over 90) are less likely to have Parkinson's.[15]

Genetic factors

Most cases of Parkinson's are sporadic (in other words, isolated incidents having no pattern). However, genetic factors are still of interest to Parkinson's researchers for two reasons:

- occasionally Parkinson's does run in families and it is important to understand why; and
- there is a theory that some people may inherit a genetic susceptibility to Parkinson's, which by itself would not cause Parkinson's but if combined with other factors may make its development more likely.

With regard to familial cases of Parkinson's, research has shown that there are some genetic mutations (changes in the composition in genes) found in these families. Research has also identified specific proteins produced by these genes, which seem to have some causal link to Parkinson's. Two of these genetic mutations are of particular interest:

- Park 1 is a gene that was identified in a study of a large Italian family, many members of which had Parkinson's. This gene produces a protein called alpha-synuclein, which is a major component of Lewy bodies (the abnormal cells that are found in the brains of people with Parkinson's). Researchers think that the accumulation of alpha-synuclein in the Lewy body is central to the development of Parkinson's. Gene mutations of this protein have not been found in sporadic Parkinson's[16]; and

• Park 2 (also known as the Parkin gene) is a gene that is found predominantly in people who have juvenile parkinsonism (which is defined as starting before the age of 21).

Genetic research has also focused on the mitochondria, which are components of the cells of the body and which are responsible for turning nutrients into energy. The theory is that some cases of Parkinson's may be transmitted through a defect in mitochondrial genes.[17]

These possible genetic links to some cases of Parkinson's are the subject of ongoing research.

Environmental factors

Researchers have looked at possible neurotoxic causes of Parkinson's and, conversely, possible neuroprotective agents that might reduce the risk of someone getting Parkinson's.

Neurotoxins

Interest in neurotoxins was kindled in the late 1970s and early 1980s by some US drug addicts who rapidly developed Parkinson's-like symptoms after taking a designer drug that was synthesized to produce similar effects to heroin. The synthesized drug was found to contain a substance called MPTP (1-methyl-4-phenyl-1,2,3,6-tetrahydropyridine), which the body converted into a specific toxin called MPP+. This toxin caused the death of the dopamine-producing neurones in the substantia nigra.[18]

Although there are unlikely to be large enough quantities of MPTP in the environment to cause Parkinson's, it is structurally similar to many other substances, such as pesticides. Parkinson's has also been associated with water from wells, rural living and farming.[19] However, these associations have not been clearly established and further research is needed.

Neuroprotection

Many researchers are interested in the role of damage from free radicals as a possible cause of Parkinson's. Free radicals are highly reactive and potentially very damaging molecules, produced by normal chemical reactions in the body or absorbed from outside sources through cigarette smoke, pollutants or prolonged exposure to sunlight. Although they last for only a very short time, they have the potential to do damage to the cells of the body during that time. Dopamine-producing cells seem to be particularly at risk from free radical generation and damage.[20]

Antioxidants, which are chemicals produced by the body or absorbed from the diet, neutralize the effects of free radicals. As a result, several antioxidants have been studied as possible neuroprotective agents and possible Parkinson's treatments. However, apart from co-enzyme Q10, evidence is lacking for the neuroprotective effect of these antioxidants.

Co-enzyme Q10 is found in every cell of the body, as well as in certain foods such as beef, soya oil, sardines, mackerel, peanuts, and organ meats including kidney, liver and heart. Co-enzyme Q10 supplements are also available. Research studies have suggested that high doses of co-enzyme Q10 can slow the progression of Parkinson's. However, although these findings are encouraging, much more research is needed.[21]

Tobacco, coffee and tea have also been of interest because it is thought they may have an ingredient that helps to protect people against Parkinson's. There is evidence that people who drink coffee or who smoke are less likely to have Parkinson's. Although the harmful effects of smoking outweigh any neuroprotective effect that cigarettes might have, researchers have studied the effects of nicotine on Parkinson's, but the results have been disappointing.[22]

Viruses

Viruses have been considered as a possible cause of Parkinson's by researchers since cases of post-encephalitic parkinsonism emerged after the encephalitis lethargica epidemic of 1916–26 (see Chapter 1). Viruses continue to be an area of research into the cause of Parkinson's. However, even if a virus were found to be a causal agent in Parkinson's, it is unlikely that the parkinsonism would be infectious.

Head injury

There are many theories about head injuries possibly causing Parkinson's; however, minor head injuries do not cause Parkinson's. Occasionally some people who have a significant head injury subsequently develop symptoms of Parkinson's, though the relationship between the two has not yet been established.

3

Symptoms

This chapter looks at some of the common Parkinson's symptoms. It is not exhaustive, and it is important that you discuss any symptoms with your doctor or Parkinson's disease nurse specialist, to help you to manage them and so that any that might have another cause can be highlighted.

If you are newly diagnosed with Parkinson's, reading about these symptoms can be frightening. Remember that each person with Parkinson's is very different, and you may not experience all of the symptoms or problems described. Each person I interviewed had different symptoms, and none of them had all of them.

Tremor

Most people instantly link Parkinson's to tremor, despite the fact that 30 per cent of people with Parkinson's don't experience it. The tremor of Parkinson's is a distinctive one known as a 'resting tremor', which tends to occur when the affected part of the body is at rest and lessens when it is being used. There are several other types of tremor that have different causes from Parkinson's (such as essential tremor – see Chapter 1).

Tremor in Parkinson's often starts in a hand or arm on one side of the body, although it can affect other parts of the body as well. Some people also feel an 'inner' tremor. Although it often remains unilateral (one-sided), sometimes tremor eventually spreads to both sides of the body. Although it can sometimes interfere with daily activities, Parkinson's tremor is often more of a nuisance than disabling. Many people find it particularly noticeable when they are in a social situation. Tiredness and any kind of stress can often exacerbate tremor.

The drug treatments for Parkinson's can help to reduce tremor, although they often can't suppress it completely. If the tremor is particularly dominant or disabling, surgery may help.

Rigidity

Rigidity, which the person with Parkinson's feels as stiffness, can cause changes in posture, and people may find they become stooped or bent over, with a tendency to bend the arms and legs at the elbows, hips and knees. Many people also experience pain, particularly in the neck, shoulders and arms.

Slowness and poverty of movement

The symptoms of slowness of movement (bradykinesia), reduced movement (hypokinesia) and inability to initiate movement (akinesia) are probably the most disabling and frustrating features of the condition.[23]

People with Parkinson's find that their movements become unco-ordinated, harder to initiate and take longer to perform. Difficulties with fine finger movements such as handwriting can be among the first symptoms to appear.

Walking and balance are often affected, often at first in subtle ways – for example, loss of arm swing while walking can be an early sign of Parkinson's. When walking, people often find that they take smaller shorter steps, which get faster as they walk (festination). There is also a tendency to shuffle because the feet are not raised as high as they used to be when walking. Stopping suddenly, turning or having to change direction can also be difficult. All of these, combined with rigidity and posture problems, can make people with Parkinson's more likely to fall. The risk of this can be increased by low blood pressure, which can be a symptom of the condition as well as a side-effect of some of the drugs used to treat Parkinson's.

Any kind of daily or nightly activity can be affected. Rising from a chair can be difficult and once in a standing position, it can be hard for the person to achieve enough balance to stand up unaided. Some people also find that when they are sitting, there is a tendency to lean to one side. Some people find it easier to sit in a chair with arms, which provides some support when they need to get up from it. Getting in and out of bed can also be a problem, as can turning over in bed, though slippery satin sheets can often make this easier.

The drugs prescribed for Parkinson's can often help with these problems, as can advice from physiotherapists and occupational therapists (see Chapter 5).

Freezing[24]

Freezing means stopping suddenly while walking or when beginning to start a movement, and then being unable to move forward again for several seconds or minutes.

People with Parkinson's describe it as feeling as if their feet are frozen or stuck to the ground, with the top half of their body wanting to move on. Freezing can also be experienced when the person is doing other activities or when starting a movement, such as moving off after rising from a chair, getting out of bed or starting to speak. Freezing when approaching doorways or lifts seems to be particularly common. There is no consistency in freezing but it tends to become worse if the person is anxious or in an unfamiliar place or loses concentration. Freezing can lead to problems with balance and falls, and some people lose confidence about going out in public places without someone else.

Why the normal sequence of movement gets interrupted is unclear. Freezing is slightly more common in people whose initial symptoms involved difficulties with gait and balance and is far more likely to happen in people who have had Parkinson's for several years and who have been treated with levodopa.

Freezing should be discussed with your doctor, who may be able to adjust your medication. A physiotherapist can advise on helpful techniques, such as marching on the spot, imagining stepping over a stick or counting 'one, two, three' to get going again.

Muscle cramps and dystonia

The rigidity together with slowness and poverty of movement can cause muscle cramps, which some people find very painful. Dystonia – sustained involuntary contractions of the muscles, which cause the affected part of the body to go into a spasm[25] – can be common. Dystonia is more likely to affect younger people with Parkinson's. It can be a symptom of Parkinson's but may also be caused by the drugs used to treat the condition. Adjustments to the drugs can sometimes help.

Tiredness[26]

Fatigue can be a common problem. People with Parkinson's have to work much harder to achieve normal, everyday tasks that someone without Parkinson's would take for granted. Activities that were previously done without thinking now require more conscious effort, which can make people very tired. Tremor and rigidity can also put particular stress on the muscles, making them work harder, often against each other, in order to initiate movement or to complete an action. As a result the muscles become tired very quickly and easily.

Slowness of movement can mean that tasks take longer to complete than they used to do. Some people, particularly if they are working, may try to complete these too quickly, resulting in tiredness and stress. Side-effects of medication that can occur with long-term use, such as fluctuations in mobility and dyskinesias, can also contribute to fatigue.

Fatigue can cause people to become less active because of the exhaustion they feel. This in turn can have an impact on a person's physical, intellectual and emotional lives as well. If the person is doing less, his or her interests decline, with resultant feelings of isolation and boredom, which in turn can lead to depression.

Sleep problems are also common in Parkinson's, caused either by symptoms or by drugs.

If fatigue is a problem, you should discuss it with your doctor. Fatigue can have other causes than Parkinson's. If Parkinson's is the reason, your fatigue may be treated through medication, although this is not always successful. Two drugs used to treat Parkinson's, amantadine (*Symmetrel*) and selegiline (*Eldepryl* and *Zelapar*) have a mild stimulant effect and may be helpful if given at low doses during the daytime. Some doctors also try drugs that promote wakefulness, such as modafinil (*Provigil*), but the long-term effects of using this type of drug treatment in people with Parkinson's is not yet fully known.

Communication problems

Although some people experience very few communication problems even after several years, about 50 per cent of those with Parkinson's do develop difficulties with speech and non-verbal communication, including facial expression and body language.

Speech may become slurred or monotonous in tone, with a lack of variation and expression in the voice; it may also be affected in its rate and rhythm and sometimes its intelligibility. There can be hesitancy or difficulty in getting the voice started, and, once a person has started talking, speech may get progressively faster. This can mean that people with Parkinson's are not readily understood by other people. Talking in a crowd or over noise and everyday activities such as using the phone may become impossible.

Facial expression and body language can also be reduced, mainly because of muscle rigidity and slowness of movement. There can be a lack of spontaneity in body language and an absence of gestures, such as nodding, and many people have difficulty making ordinary facial expressions such as frowning and smiling.

These communication problems can have a profound effect on an affected person's relationships. They can also lead to incorrect assumptions being made – one example, which is often cited by people I have talked to, is being thought to be drunk because of the slurred speech and unsteady balance. Carrying one of the Parkinson's Alert Cards (M14) produced by the Parkinson's Disease Society can help in these situations or in an emergency when you are unable to communicate clearly. Drugs can sometimes help improve speech problems, as can a speech and language therapist (see Chapter 5).

Handwriting problems

Difficulties with handwriting can be one of the earliest signs of Parkinson's and are generally caused by tremor and lack of co-ordination. Many people with Parkinson's find that when they start to write, the size of their handwriting is normal but as they write across the page, their writing becomes smaller and smaller (micrographia). Some people also find their writing becomes spidery and difficult to read, which can make it harder to write a consistent signature on cheques and official documents.

There are various ways of overcoming problems with handwriting, such as using a felt-tip pen or a thick or padded pen or pencil, wearing a weighted cuff to help dampen down the tremor, and using a non-slip mat or a clipboard to prevent the paper from slipping. An occupational therapist can advise further (see Chapter 5).

Information technology, such as computers, the internet and e-mail, also offer alternative ways of communicating.

Drooling and difficulty in swallowing

Drooling – having saliva pooling and trickling from the mouth – can be a common and distressing problem. Excess saliva is not the reason. It occurs because the automatic tendency to swallow is slowed down in Parkinson's. Changes in posture caused by the condition can also be a contributory factor. The head tends to be held tilted forwards, causing saliva to accumulate in the front of the mouth. Instead of being swallowed, the saliva can leak out of the mouth especially if the person has poor lip closure, which means the lips do not seal tightly.

Swallowing problems are not common in the early stages of Parkinson's, but can be experienced by some people who have had the condition for several years.

Drooling and swallowing difficulties are generally connected and should be discussed with your doctor – adjustment of your medication may help. Speech and language therapists may also be able to help (see Chapter 5).

Bowel problems

Constipation is very common and can have several causes. Slowness of movement and rigidity can affect the bowel muscles and this, combined with lack of movement, can mean that the bowel doesn't get the stimuli it needs to function properly. Some people with Parkinson's have problems with chewing and swallowing food and so don't eat enough fibre (found in many vegetables, fruits and grains). Some medications used to treat Parkinson's, particularly anticholinergic drugs, can also worsen constipation.

Some people may also have problems emptying the bowel. Because of Parkinson's, it can be difficult to brace the abdominal muscles to assist bowel emptying, and the anal sphincter, which controls the passage of faeces out of the body, may not relax at the right time to allow the stool to be passed easily. Some people actually get a paradoxical contraction of the sphincter when trying to empty the bowel – the anus tightens when they think they are relaxing it.

Increasing your intake of fluids and fibre-rich foods, as well as taking more exercise, may help (though bear in mind that too much bulk from fibre can actually increase constipation). If exercise is difficult for you, ask your doctor to refer you to a physiotherapist or dietician (see Chapters 5 and 9).

In extreme cases, a laxative might help, but you should not use one without consulting your doctor, because long-term use of laxatives can worsen constipation and damage the bowel.

Skin and sweating problems[27]

Some people with Parkinson's find that their skin and scalp may become greasy and scaly. This is because Parkinson's can cause the glands in the skin to overproduce a secretion called sebum, which keeps the skin supple and protects it. This is sometimes called seborrhoea. The drugs used to treat Parkinson's can improve this problem. Washing the skin with a neutral soap can also help.

Excessive sweating is another problem, particularly at night. This can be caused by Parkinson's itself and also by some of the medications, such as levodopa. However, some drugs, such as anticholinergics, can make people sweat too little. Adjustments to the drugs can help in some cases.

Personal experiences

Graham

Graham, who has had Parkinson's for 12 years, was diagnosed at 52, and at the time was a senior bank manager. His handwriting had always been bad but it started to get smaller and he found he made a lot of mistakes when typing. His GP, whom he knew well, took 10 minutes to diagnose Parkinson's and then referred him to a specialist, who confirmed the diagnosis.

Graham and his wife Lesley didn't know anything about Parkinson's at the time, and the images they had in their head or from books they looked at were of old people shaking or sitting in wheelchairs. 'On the whole it hasn't turned out to be as bad as we initially thought it might be, and we have learnt to deal with it. It is important not to let Parkinson's take over your whole life and stop you from doing the things you like doing.'

Graham's day fluctuates and each one is different. His biggest problem is with his voice. He always spoke quickly, but his Parkinson's makes him speak even faster, sometimes making it hard for people to understand what he is saying. Speech and language therapy has helped, with techniques such as using smaller words and adopting the right posture when speaking to stop the diaphragm from getting squashed and affecting the voice. Graham also has a computer and uses e-mail extensively.

Graham didn't start medication when he was first diagnosed. Since starting on it, he has changed his drug regimen several times. The drugs take some time to work so deadlines can be tricky and planning is important. He also experiences 'on–offs' as a side-effect (see Chapter 6). If he is 'off', he can't always speak when someone telephones.

At times he feels constrained because he has to take more precautions if he goes out on his own, and he always carries a mobile phone so he can contact someone if he gets into difficulties. He also takes two wallet-sized cards about Parkinson's, one with a list of his drugs, and the other an alert card, which helps him if he goes 'off' in a public place and is unable to talk. 'I find if you have something that identifies you as having Parkinson's, people are more willing to help.'

Graham told his employers immediately that he had Parkinson's, and he continued to work for four years before taking early retirement. He and his wife also told their adult children, who were very supportive.

Although Graham's speech problems prevent him from doing as much committee work as he used to, he still acts in an advisory capacity to the Scouts and has travelled to Russia to celebrate a Russian Scouts jamboree. He has also become involved with his local branch of the Parkinson's Disease Society, a source of great support and reassurance. When Lesley retired, shortly after Graham, they agreed they wouldn't just slump in front of the television, so one of the first things they did was take a holiday touring the USA by train.

'I am very lucky because of the support my family give me and the financial security I have from my long service with the bank. Financial stability makes a big difference to coping. Because of my banking background, I am concerned that people don't always know how to access the help that they are entitled to. Our branch of the Parkinson's Disease Society has a community support worker, who has managed to help many members obtain benefits. I think the forms are very complicated and so much depends on how people answer the questions. You always need to make sure that you put down what things are like for you on a bad day.'

Rosemary

Rosemary, aged 67, has had Parkinson's for seven years. She was diagnosed after noticing her main symptom, a shaking leg. Her doctor referred her to a specialist, who asked her to walk and do things with her fingers and then ordered a brain scan before telling her that she had Parkinson's.

Parkinson's affects Rosemary in many different ways. 'The main symptoms I experience at the moment are tremor, stiffness, tiredness and slowness of movement. The tremor makes daily tasks difficult and causes me anxiety when I'm with other people as I become embarrassed, which exacerbates the tremor even more. I have problems with my handwriting and I have had signatures challenged in the bank as a result. The stiffness means that I am slow to "get going". Daily tasks take much longer than they used to. The stiffness can get worse and then my body starts to freeze up. I might be rooted to the spot, which I find scary. I often feel tired and need to take frequent naps to get through the day and enable me to complete my daily tasks in between.'

Her husband Peter helps her with some daily tasks such as showering and getting in and out of the bath. She also has small pieces of equipment, such as handrails, which can be useful. Cooking can be a problem because she can't do anything that involves using an oven. She tends to prepare the food and then hands over to Peter, who enjoys cooking and describes himself as 'chief cook and bottle-washer'.

As soon as she was diagnosed, Rosemary started on medication with ropinirole, and she now takes several drugs. Before she retired, Rosemary worked in an office and before that as a telephonist. She continued to work for a while after her diagnosis but wanted to leave before she started making mistakes. 'It was about the time when Jill Dando, the television presenter, was murdered and I thought "life's too precious" and decided to give up work.

Making decisions like this is difficult but once you've made it, it becomes easier – but you need to be the one to make the decision.'

Although frustrated by her loss of independence – she does not go out unaccompanied and gave up driving some years ago – Rosemary keeps very busy. She enjoys sewing, knitting, and jigsaw puzzles, as well as sequence old-time dancing, supported by Peter.

'I think you should be positive about Parkinson's – it lives with me, I don't live with it. Although it's difficult, Parkinson's isn't all doom and gloom. It has made me realize what I really value – the patience and understanding of my husband, family and friends. I won't give things up and I still need a challenge.'

4

Diagnosis

One of the most frustrating aspects of Parkinson's is the fact that there are currently no definitive medical tests to prove that someone has it.

The only conclusive evidence is the presence of microscopic deposits called Lewy bodies that appear inside damaged neurones (nerve cells) in the substantia nigra, the part of the brain affected in Parkinson's. However, these deposits cannot be used as markers for Parkinson's when making a diagnosis in life because they can only be seen when the brains of people with Parkinson's are examined after death. Lewy bodies are not found in other forms of parkinsonism, apart from dementia with Lewy bodies, where the extent and pattern of distribution is quite different from that seen in Parkinson's (see Chapter 1).

Diagnosis is usually made by the doctor, who takes a medical history and performs a clinical examination.

Who diagnoses?

Because of the complicated, individual nature of Parkinson's and its treatment, the Parkinson's Disease Society and the European Parkinson's Disease Association both recommend that all people with Parkinson's should be referred to a specialist doctor who has a particular interest in Parkinson's. GPs play a very important, indeed invaluable, role in the long-term care of people with Parkinson's. However, referral to a specialist is important because diagnosis relies on medical history and clinical examination and also because the symptoms of Parkinson's can have other causes.

The specialist will also have a greater knowledge of the treatments and management options currently available – important because of the individuality of Parkinson's symptoms and the response to treatment that different people experience. Also, as Parkinson's progresses, treatments often have to be reviewed and adjusted.

Many specialists run special Parkinson's disease clinics or work closely with a multidisciplinary team, such as Parkinson's disease nurse specialists and therapists. Although these types of services can also be provided via the GP, access and cross-referral (that is, referral from one health professional to another) can often be easier if you are on a specialist's list.

There are two types of doctors who tend to specialize in Parkinson's – neurologists and geriatricians.

Neurologists specialize in diseases of the nervous system – the brain, spine and nerves. Not all neurologists specialize in Parkinson's. Those who do have a particular interest in movement disorders – a group of conditions, including Parkinson's, that affect a person's ability to start and control movement. People of all ages can be referred to a neurologist, but if you are a younger person with Parkinson's, this is the type of specialist you are most likely to see.

Geriatricians are consultant physicians with a special interest in the care of the elderly, usually defined as people aged over 65. Because Parkinson's is a condition that is more common in older people, many people with Parkinson's will see a geriatrician. Many older people with Parkinson's also have other conditions, such as diabetes, stroke or arthritis, that can complicate treatment and care. Geriatricians tend to have a good knowledge of these other conditions and how they may interact with Parkinson's. As a principle of practice, geriatricians also tend to work in multidisciplinary teams.

Making the diagnosis

The doctor will ask you about your symptoms and examine you, looking at three key areas:

- establishing that symptoms of Parkinson's are present;
- excluding any other possible causes; and
- finding supporting evidence of Parkinson's.

Slowness of movement (bradykinesia) is one of the first symptoms your doctor will look for, along with any indications of muscular rigidity, resting tremor or postural instability.

Blood tests and scans may be used to rule out other conditions, such as tumours and strokes. Once other causes have been eliminated, the doctor may make a tentative diagnosis of Parkinson's but will look for supporting evidence.

Response to the drugs used to treat Parkinson's is one such indicator. People with Parkinson's generally have a good response, while people with other forms of parkinsonism generally do not respond to or respond less well to the drugs. To gauge this, some doctors will prescribe particular drugs and ask you to come back in a few weeks' time to review what effect they are having on your symptoms.

Others will carry out an 'acute dopaminergic drug challenge test' in the clinic – you will be given either levodopa or apomorphine (two drugs used to treat Parkinson's), with assessments of your motor function being made before and after each dose. A positive response to the drug provides further evidence that you have Parkinson's. However, response to drugs is not an infallible method of determining Parkinson's because sometimes people with idiopathic Parkinson's disease have a poor response to the drugs and, conversely, people who subsequently turn out to have a different form of parkinsonism can respond well initially to the drugs.

Sometimes time can be a factor in making a diagnosis, particularly in cases where the diagnosis is uncertain at the first meeting. Because Parkinson's usually starts slowly, the symptoms may be more apparent when a few months have lapsed, making diagnosis easier.

Neuroimaging

Neuroimaging studies the brain and other parts of the nervous system. There are two main types of neuroimaging – structural imaging and functional imaging. Sometimes some sorts of imaging may be used as part of the diagnostic process, though none of them can definitely diagnose Parkinson's.

Structural imaging

Structural imaging allows the doctor to identify parts of the brain such as blood vessels, grey matter and white matter. Although structural images can provide good details of how a person's brain looks, they cannot give a very detailed picture of how the brain is functioning. Examples include computed tomography or computerized tomography (CT) or computed axial tomography (CAT), and magnetic resonance imaging (MRI).

CT scans are a more sophisticated type of X-ray. A conventional X-ray gives a two-dimensional image of the outline of bones and organs. A CT scan, aided by computer technology, can pass a series of X-rays through the body at slightly different angles to produce detailed cross-sections or 'slices' of organs and tissues. These slices can also be combined to make a three-dimensional image of the part of the body being scanned. CT scans are generally used to detect tumours and strokes.

MRI scanning has been used since the early 1980s to provide images of internal organs and structures. It is particularly useful for detecting brain tumours and is often used to help confirm a diagnosis of multiple sclerosis. MRI can also show structural changes or abnormalities within the basal ganglia, the part of the brain where dopamine cells are made. It may be used in cases where the diagnosis is unclear in order to detect changes in the brain that are more typical of multiple system atrophy (MSA) or progressive supranuclear palsy (PSP).

Functional imaging

Functional imaging provides pictures of how the brain is working and allows doctors to investigate functions of the brain, such as blood flow and activity of cells in certain areas of the brain.

Radionuclide scanning is a commonly used type of functional imaging. Radionuclides are harmless radioactive substances. In radionuclide scanning, a radionuclide tracer is introduced into the body. The tracer binds to particular organs or tissues, which are then imaged. Different tissues take up different radionuclides, so the particular radionuclide used depends on what part of the body is being scanned. A counter placed outside the body detects the radiation emitted by the radionuclide and sends this information to a computer, which then converts the information into images. A radionuclide scan will usually show the parts of the body as areas of colour of varying intensity. Where the colour is intense, the tissue in that area is very active. Where there is low intensity in colour, the tissue is less active. Therefore this kind of scan can be very useful for showing areas of abnormal activity in the body. Types of radionuclide scanning of particular interest in the diagnosis of parkinsonism are single-photon emission computed tomography (SPECT) and positron emission tomography (PET).These are sometimes used when a diagnosis is difficult to make.

SPECT was developed in the 1970s. Although at first it was used exclusively for research purposes, it is now more widely applied in medicine and is available in most large hospitals in the UK. SPECT is of particular interest in the diagnosis of parkinsonism because it can be used with two iodine-based tracers, ^{123}I-beta-CIT and ^{123}I-FP-CIT (also known as DaTSCAN), to provide an image of the activity of dopamine cells in the substantia nigra. These radionuclides bind to the dopamine cells and emit particles, known as photons, which the scanner can detect; the scanner can then produce an image of varying brightness depending on how active these cells are. An image that is not very bright indicates that the dopamine cells are not functioning as well as they should be. However, the SPECT scan cannot determine what form of parkinsonism the person has, although when used with DaTSCAN it can distinguish between essential tremor (where dopamine loss will not be seen on the scan) and other forms of parkinsonism.

PET scanning also uses radionuclides to trace activity of cells and tissues in the body but, unlike SPECT, it uses a tracer called ^{18}F-6-fluorodopa (^{18}F-dopa) to detect particles called positrons. The tracer is taken up by dopamine cells in the substantia nigra, and the rate of accumulation of ^{18}F-dopa, which is dependent on the activity of the cells, is then measured by the PET scanner. The fewer active cells there are, the less the ^{18}F-dopa will be detected by the scanner. Although PET is a useful means of measuring the loss of dopamine cells in Parkinson's, it is seldom used to make a diagnosis because reduced uptake of ^{18}F-dopa is also found in people with multiple system atrophy (MSA).

Moreover, sometimes PET and SPECT scans can appear normal in people with Parkinson's at diagnosis. There are also only about five PET scanners in the UK and the technique is so expensive that PET scanning is generally only used for research purposes.

Advances in diagnosis

There are several research studies currently under way.

Altropane, a new chemical imaging agent, is currently being researched at the Harvard Medical School and Massachusetts General Hospital in the USA. This has the potential to diagnose Parkinson's more accurately and at an earlier stage than is currently possible.

Dr Kay Double and her team at the Prince of Wales Medical Research Institute in Sydney, Australia, have developed a blood test that can detect Parkinson's soon after the symptoms begin to show. This test is still at a very experimental stage but it also has the potential, if successful, to identify people with Parkinson's before the development of symptoms.

The Michael J. Fox Foundation for Parkinson's Research in the USA announced a $US2 million research programme in 2002 for the development or validation of conclusive diagnostic tests or biomarkers for Parkinson's disease. Several grants have since been awarded as a result. See the Foundation's website for more information – <http://www.michaeljfox.org>.

Coping with the diagnosis

A diagnosis of Parkinson's is a life-changing event and initial reactions vary tremendously. The time of diagnosis is often a very difficult one. Even though the symptoms may be mild and well controlled at this stage, it is natural to have fears about the future. Give yourself time to come to terms with having Parkinson's and don't rush into making decisions. Gather the information that you need to help you to understand Parkinson's so you can make informed decisions about the future. Depression is very common in Parkinson's, particularly at this stage, and it is important to seek help from your doctor if you are struggling emotionally to cope with the diagnosis. (See Chapter 10 for more information about the psychological and emotional impact.)

Research has shown that the way the diagnosis is given to you, as well as the support and information provided at this stage, can make all the difference to how you subsequently cope. Unfortunately, experiences seem to vary enormously. Some people I talked to felt that their diagnosis had been given to them in a sympathetic and understanding way. The doctor had used language that they could understand and was willing to answer any questions. In addition, they had been provided with as much information as they felt they needed and referred to other sources of information, such as a Parkinson's disease nurse specialist, a key worker or the Parkinson's Disease Society. Others, however, felt that the telling of their diagnosis was not handled well and the doctor had imparted the diagnosis abruptly, using technical terms that they found difficult to understand. Furthermore, no information on Parkinson's or contact details were provided, leaving them feeling very isolated. The stress of coping with the diagnosis was compounded by the fact that they had to find their own information or support groups.

Support and information

It is to be hoped that communication of the diagnosis is improving. In recent years, medical schools have placed much more emphasis on the teaching of communication skills as part of a doctor's training. If you feel that the telling of your diagnosis was inadequate or that you were not given the necessary information or support you need, don't despair. Help is available.

The Parkinson's Disease Society has a wide range of information materials about Parkinson's and related subjects, including specific resources for newly diagnosed people and their families. Many of these can be downloaded from their website or ordered through the post. If you have any questions about Parkinson's or you want to talk to someone about how you feel, the Parkinson's Disease Society advisory line staff can help you further. There are also regional staff across the UK, who can provide you with information about what is available in your local area. This might include local branches, Young Parkinson's Support Network (YPSN, formerly known as YAPP&Rs) groups if you are younger, and community support workers who visit people at home to provide support and information (see Useful addresses).

The European Parkinson's Disease Association also has a wealth of information on their website which you might find helpful. This includes personal accounts and links to other Parkinson's sources (see Useful addresses).

If there is a Parkinson's disease nurse specialist in your area, she or he can also be a vital source of information and support (see Chapter 5).

Don't be surprised either if your feelings fluctuate from day to day or if it takes you some time to adjust – some people say it took them a number of years. Give yourself as much time as you need and remember that help is available if you need it. Living with Parkinson's isn't always easy but the people quoted in this book demonstrate that it is possible to survive a diagnosis of Parkinson's. The knowledge, understanding and treatment of Parkinson's is also improving all the time, providing hope for the future.

Whom do I tell?

This is a very personal decision and only you know what is best for you. However, it is a good idea to tell at least one person close to you so that you have someone to talk to.

Most people I interviewed had decided to be open about their Parkinson's from the start and felt this was the best approach. Most people said that their family and friends were very supportive but some people did find it difficult to deal with, reacting badly and being unable to provide them with the support they needed. The flip-side of this is that some people found that friends or acquaintances that they weren't expecting to be particularly interested or supportive responded very positively and helped them immensely.

Personal experience

Anne was diagnosed with Parkinson's nine years ago at the age of 53. At the time she was a secretary in a branch of the civil service. A keen tap dancer, she noticed when she was dancing that there were little things that were not quite right with her feet, that she had a tremor in her leg and arm at times, and that sometimes she found putting on make-up difficult.

She went to see the GP mainly because of the tremor. The doctor was very reassuring, thought it might be stress, and prescribed tranquillizers to try to see if they stopped the tremor. When they didn't, she was referred a neurologist, who diagnosed her with Parkinson's.

'My immediate reaction was relief at knowing what was wrong. However, I then looked up Parkinson's in a medical book and wept for two days. Prior to diagnosis, my attitude was ostrich-like and I didn't look anything up. My approach was to carry on with life as I had always lived it and not to give up. When I went to work the next day I told everyone that I had it. I felt people would find out anyway. Most didn't believe it as I didn't look any different.'

Paul, Anne's husband, was reassured about Parkinson's because one of his colleagues had had Parkinson's and was still doing his job. Anne also knew a woman with Parkinson's who worked at the same place as her. 'I was encouraged by how she coped with the condition and the fact that you couldn't really tell that she had Parkinson's. However, her approach was quite different from mine.

She hadn't told many people that she had it and had preferred to keep it to herself.'

Anne carried on working for two and a half years after her diagnosis and then retired. 'I could have gone on longer but an opportunity to take early retirement came up. I also wanted to leave work while I was still doing the job properly. I did wonder if I was doing the right thing but I knew I wouldn't just sit in a chair.' She has always been an independent person with lots of hobbies, such as badminton and dancing, which she keeps up. However, she finds she does less on her own these days and since Paul retired in 2003 she rarely drives.

Anne and Paul have a son and two daughters, who have always been very supportive. They are particularly proud of the fact that two of their children and one daughter's partner have run the London Marathon, raising over £5,000 for the Parkinson's Disease Society. Anne's sister has also become involved with the support group in her local area. Paul says that the openness about Anne's Parkinson's also meant that when his company closed, the Parkinson's Disease Society received a contribution from the company's welfare fund.

Anne says, 'I have tried to live my life as I have always done. I have carried on and proved that you can. I feel there are benefits in being open about having Parkinson's and I have obtained help and assistance that I might not have had if we had kept it to ourselves. I also get a lot from meeting others at the support groups.'

5

Help available

Although at present there is no cure for Parkinson's, there are treatments to help control the symptoms and to manage any particular problems. These include drugs, surgery, allied health disciplines (such as physiotherapy, speech and language therapy, and occupational therapy), community care services and self-help. Drugs, surgery and self-help are discussed in Chapters 6, 7 and 11 respectively. This chapter provides an overview of health and social care professionals or services that can help you manage your Parkinson's.

Understanding and knowledge of these areas can help you to make informed choices about your treatment. Usually, a multidisciplinary approach (many different disciplines working together to provide care) is recommended to ensure that you retain your independence and have the best possible quality of life.

Medical professionals

General practitioner

Your GP will be central to your long-term care. GPs usually work with a team, which may include practice nurses, district nurses, health visitors, therapists and counsellors. Many of the people I interviewed had a very good relationship with their GP and said that he or she was an invaluable support to them and was always willing to talk to them and advise them. GPs and specialists often work closely together.

Specialists

Specialists involved with Parkinson's tend to be either neurologists (specializing in the brain, spine and nerves) or geriatricians (consultant physicians with a particular interest in care of the elderly). Specialists often run Parkinson's clinics that involve many other health professionals, including doctors in their team, Parkinson's disease nurse specialists, and therapists. To see a specialist, you need a referral from your GP, even if you go privately.

Parkinson's disease nurse specialists

Parkinson's disease nurse specialists are registered general nurses (RGNs) who specialize in Parkinson's and its treatment. They work mainly in hospitals, alongside specialists, although some are also now employed by primary care trusts.

Although the number of Parkinson's disease nurse specialists is growing, they are not yet available in every area. Their role varies but it is broadly to provide support and information to people with Parkinson's on a wide range of issues, from advice about medication to support if you have to go to hospital.

Other nurses

Several other kinds of nurses may be involved in your care, including community nurses, practice nurses and health visitors.

Allied health professionals

Other disciplines include physiotherapy, speech and language therapy, occupational therapy, dietetics and podiatry. Practitioners of these disciplines are often grouped together under the umbrella term 'allied health professionals'. Early referral is usually recommended, and ideally you should make sure that the health professional you see has some experience of people with Parkinson's.

Physiotherapists

Since Parkinson's is a movement disorder, people can gain considerable benefit from contact with physiotherapists, even on a short-term or occasional basis. Physiotherapists may be able to help you with any mobility problems such walking, sitting down, standing up and turning over in bed, enabling you to maintain as much independence as possible. They may also help with the characteristic stiff muscles and joints of Parkinson's, as well as with freezing and preventing falls.

You usually need a referral from your GP, specialist or Parkinson's disease nurse specialist. In some places you can refer yourself at the local hospital or community health clinic. You can also see a physiotherapist privately.

Speech and language therapists

Speech and language therapists can help with many typical problems of Parkinson's, including those with speech, non-verbal communication, eating and swallowing as well as drooling. Therapists may suggest breathing and postural techniques and other exercises to help to improve communication, along with tips on making particular daily activities – such as talking on the telephone – easier to manage. They can also give useful advice to carers.

Referral is often via your GP, specialist or Parkinson's disease nurse specialist, although in many places you can refer yourself to an NHS speech and language therapist via your local hospital or health centre. Some speech and language therapists also work in private practice.

Occupational therapists

An occupational therapist can suggest ways to make it is easier for you to carry out everyday activities such as washing, dressing, cooking, housework and turning over in bed, as well as ways to make the home and work environments safer and easier – this might mean simply rearranging the furniture or it might involve adaptations ranging from grab rails on stairs to a walk-in shower in the bathroom. She or he may also offer practical advice on ways to cope with particular symptoms that you are finding difficult, such as fatigue or handwriting changes.

Your GP, specialist or Parkinson's disease nurse specialist can refer you, or in some areas you can refer yourself by contacting your local social services department. Some occupational therapists also work in private practice.

Dieticians

No special diet is required for people with Parkinson's, apart from a normal healthy diet with plenty of fruit and vegetables. However, Parkinson's can cause certain problems where advice from a dietician is invaluable. Such problems include constipation, swallowing problems – especially if you have lost weight or are malnourished as a result – and weight increase, especially if this is because of immobility or lack of regular exercise.

Some people also find that having foods rich in protein at the same time as their drugs can interfere with the absorption of the medication. If this is a problem for you, it is important that you don't reduce or cut out protein altogether as it is a vital ingredient in the diet. A dietician can advise you on ways of overcoming this problem, such as protein redistribution diets, whereby most of the daily recommended dietary protein is taken in the evening.

Referral to an NHS dietician is usually via your GP, specialist or Parkinson's disease nurse specialist. You can also see a dietician on a private basis but it is important if you do to make sure you see a registered dietician – registered dieticians have the letters RD after their name.

(Note that 'new-age' special diets, supplements and vitamins are constantly being touted as 'cures' or treatments for all kinds of health problems. Many of the claims made are without substance. It is very important to seek advice from your doctor before trying any of these diets or taking supplements or vitamins, because some can interfere with Parkinson's medication.)

Podiatrists[28]

Referral to a podiatrist (also known as a chiropodist) is important for those with Parkinson's, as foot problems are common because of the trouble people have with walking, posture and cramps. Many people, particularly if they are older, also have conditions such as diabetes and arthritis, in which care of the feet is vital in order to prevent serious health problems.

Parkinson's tremor, difficulties with fine movements of the fingers and problems with bending over can make cutting toenails more difficult. Muscle cramps and dystonia (involuntary muscle contractions) can also create pressure problems on parts of the feet not designed to withstand such strain. This can cause the toes to curl in a claw-like way. Sometimes the ankle can also turn inwards and put pressure on the outside of the foot. The big toe can also stick up and rub on the top of the shoe. These muscle cramps and dystonias can be caused by Parkinson's itself, but are often connected to Parkinson's medication, so adjustment of the medication can sometimes help.

Slowness of movement can cause circulation problems, which result in swelling of the feet. Circulation of the blood relies on movement of the legs and contractions of the leg muscles to propel the blood in the veins upwards to the heart. If a person doesn't move very much, the veins can become congested, resulting in some fluid leaking out and accumulating in the tissue of the feet and ankles. This effect, called oedema, usually builds up during the day and diminishes overnight. It is often called 'postural oedema' because it is the effect of gravity, as the person stands, that causes the accumulation of fluid around the ankles. The swelling is usually mild, but the legs may feel heavy, and putting on tight shoes may be difficult. These problems can be helped by Parkinson's drug treatment, especially if it enables the person to become more mobile. Diuretics (drugs that increase the amount of urine) can also sometimes help. If you are less mobile and oedema is a problem for you, lying flat with the legs slightly raised for an hour or so can help dissipate the excess fluid.

Although your doctor will play a key role in any foot problems described above, the podiatrist will also be vital in the treatment of these problems. The podiatrist can also provide you with general advice on care of your feet and the treatment of other foot problems, such as corns, calluses and in-growing toenails. The podiatrist can also advise on othoses (tailor-made devices such as shoe inserts or arch supports), which are used to improve gait and alleviate foot and leg pain.

Referral is via your GP or a member of his or her primary care team, your specialist or your Parkinson's disease nurse specialist; alternatively, you can see a podiatrist privately.

Pharmacists

Coping with medication, especially if you have a complex regimen involving several drugs, can be one of the most challenging aspects of having Parkinson's. This can be further complicated if you are being treated for other conditions as well. Your local pharmacist can advise you on ways of managing your medication.

Community pharmacists

Your local pharmacist can help with questions about your medication – for example, what to do if you have difficulty swallowing tablets; when to crush and when not to crush tablets; whether to take them before, with or after food; possible side-effects; and any interactions with other drugs. The pharmacist can also advise you on the suitability of any over-the-counter medicines (for example, to treat the symptoms of a cold) or complementary therapy products such as herbal treatments, homoeopathic medicines and aromatherapy oils. It is important to check that these will not interact with your prescribed medicine.

All pharmacists keep a computer record of patients' medication, which can include details of any allergies and acts as an extra safeguard against unwanted side-effects and adverse interactions if you are taking several drugs on a long-term basis. Make sure your pharmacist knows and records anything you are taking.

Pharmacists can also advise whether you need to pay prescription charges and, if you do, how you can obtain a prepayment certificate (or 'season ticket') for medications that you need on a regular basis.

Community pharmacists can also provide you with advice on general health matters. Don't be afraid to ask them. Remember that however difficult or embarrassing you find this, they are there to help and you won't be the first to ask! All information you share with them will be confidential.

If you are admitted to hospital, the hospital pharmacist also plays a role in your care, working with medical and nursing staff to ensure that you are given the most appropriate treatment while in hospital.

Primary Care Trusts

Primary Care Trusts are a key part of the NHS and are responsible for managing health services in local areas. They ensure that there are enough services in the area they cover and that all health services are provided and accessible. They also have a responsibility for ensuring that health and social care systems work together to the patients' benefit. Services covered by Primary Care Trusts include GPs, hospitals, dentists, opticians, pharmacies, mental health services, walk-in centres, patient transport (including accident and emergency services), and population screening. Your local phone directory should have details of your local Primary Care Trust.

All Primary Care Trusts have Patient Advice and Liaison Services (PALS), which aim to:

• provide you with help and information on local health care services and support agencies;

- offer practical advice to help to resolve difficulties that you may have when using an NHS service or if you don't know how to access a service; and
- give you a say in your own care and how your local services operate.

Patient Advice and Liaison Services also provide information to the Primary Care Trust board about concerns that patients have expressed about services so that problems can be solved and services improved. They can't get involved in formal complaints but they can advise you about the NHS complaints system, which includes local Independent Complaint Advocacy Services (ICAS), which can support people making a formal complaint. Your local Primary Care Trust, GP surgery or hospital should be able to provide you with contact details for your local Patient Advice and Liaison Service.

Day hospitals and rehabilitation centres

Day hospitals and rehabilitation centres may house a pool of health professionals such as physiotherapists, occupational therapists, speech and language therapists, nurses and doctors, with links to others including dieticians, podiatrists, psychologists, counsellors and social service teams. They also provide support to carers.

The benefits are that instead of having to see each member of the team separately, you can see them all in one place on the same day, so that ideally an overall programme of care is developed to meet your individual needs.

They also often provide group activities and talks, which give you an opportunity to meet other people.

Referral criteria depend on your local area. Your GP, specialist or Parkinson's disease nurse specialist should be able to advise you further.

Social services

With advances in treatment, many people with Parkinson's live comfortably and independently at home for years. However, as Parkinson's progresses, some people find that they need extra help to enable them to cope more easily at home – for example, with housework or with personal care tasks such as washing and dressing or advice about adaptations to the home.

Your particular needs (and those of your carer, if necessary) will be established by way of a community care assessment, generally in your own home. Even if you don't feel you need any extra help at the moment, planning for the future is important.

Equipment

Although equipment can be useful, it is not always the answer and can be very expensive. Also, because Parkinson's is such an individual condition, what suits one person may not suit another.

Before purchasing any type of equipment, you should obtain an assessment from the relevant therapist, who can assess your needs and make recommendations so that you don't spend considerable sums on unsuitable equipment.

An occupational therapist would advise on activities of daily living such as washing, bathing, dressing, eating, reading and leisure activities.

A physiotherapist would advise on mobility problems inside and outside the house. This is complicated, however, by the fact that in some places an occupational therapist will also advise on equipment such as wheelchairs.

A speech and language therapist would advise on any problems to do with communication and also on swallowing problems. However, an occupational therapist is more likely to advise on problems to do with handwriting.

Another source of advice and information on equipment matters is the Disabled Living Foundation, a charity that specializes in providing practical advice and information on equipment to help disabled people (see Useful addresses).

Who pays for the equipment depends on the type of equipment in question, your particular circumstances (for example, whether you are on benefits) and the funding that is available in your local area or from other sources. The therapist, your GP, your hospital doctor or your Parkinson's disease nurse specialist should be able to tell you what is available.

Adaptations to your home

You may find that as your Parkinson's progresses, you need to make adaptations to your home, such as adding a ramp to your front door, refitting a bathroom or fitting a stair lift. Again, do first seek the advice of an occupational therapist, who can help assess your difficulties and recommend accordingly.

Care and Repair is an organization that helps elderly and disabled people to live in their own homes independently for as long as possible. They produce a useful guide, *In Good Repair*, which talks about repairs, adaptations, funding and finding a reliable builder or tradesman.

Advice can also be obtained from the Disabled Living Foundation, an organization that provides information on all kinds of equipment for people with disabilities, and the Centre for Accessible Environments, an organization that advises on making buildings environmentally accessible for people who are elderly or disabled (see Useful addresses).

Sometimes, if the Parkinson's is very advanced, people need to consider alternative accommodation, such as sheltered housing or residential or nursing homes.

Voluntary organizations

A voluntary organization or charity operates independently from government or business in the UK. Such organizations usually operate for a particular purpose, are self-governing, self-funding (through donations and fundraising initiatives) and not-for-profit. Although many have paid staff, they often also rely heavily on volunteers to help them run their activities.

Some voluntary organizations can provide invaluable help and support, such as the Parkinson's Disease Society, Help the Aged, Age Concern, AbilityNet, RADAR – to name but a few. For more details, contact The National Council for Voluntary Organizations or your local reference library.

Have a look at the Useful addresses section of this book (see page 120), which lists a range of organizations that I hope may be of use.

Personal experiences

Most of the people I spoke to derived great benefit from contact with the services and professionals described in this chapter. Waiting times were a problem for some, although others said that they had not had to wait very long at all. Unfortunately, since the demand for these services does vary, what is available differs depending on your area.

Anne

Anne feels that she has been very lucky in the medical support that she has had since she was diagnosed with Parkinson's. Every four months she sees her specialist or specialist nurse, whose support she especially values. She also sees her GP, who is very supportive. Anne has also been referred for speech and language therapy and occupational therapy. She picked up lots of tips from the Parkinson's Disease Society's magazine – for example, that satin sheets make turning in bed easier. She saw the speech therapist because she had problems with food not going down when she swallowed. The therapist was very helpful but had a waiting list of 10 months, which Anne would have found very difficult had the problem not eased.

Rosemary

Rosemary has always felt that she has had plenty of back-up. Her GP referred her to a specialist immediately although she then had to wait six months for the appointment, which was hard. When she went to see her GP following her diagnosis, she had plenty of time for her and referred her to the Parkinson's disease nurse specialist, who provided helpful information. She also had a visit from a local Parkinson's Disease Society community support worker. Her previous specialist has retired so she now has a new one, whom she sees every six months. The previous specialist had a Parkinson's clinic where she could see all members of the multidisciplinary team in one go. She hopes the new one will continue with this as she thinks it was brilliant.

Di

Di, who was 44 when she was diagnosed eight years ago, was referred to a local rehabilitation day centre for people with long-term conditions because of her balance problems. She found arriving on patient transport a bit of an ordeal, mainly because having been a midwife she found it difficult to adopt a 'patient's' role. However, once she was there, everyone was very friendly and she was given a course of physiotherapy and had a home visit from the occupational therapist, Liz, who provided small pieces of equipment, such as handrails or grips by the bed and on the stairs.

She struck up a friendship with Liz, who felt that there was very little local support for people with Parkinson's and wanted to develop something. So, with the help of the Parkinson's Disease Society, they set up the Billericay and Wickford Support Group. To begin with the group met in the day centre's sitting room but they have had to move to a larger venue because there are now about 45 members. Di says that helping other people through this group has given her back her confidence and provided her with a new purpose. She has been particularly delighted to find that some people who had been very reluctant to come to the meetings have blossomed through the contact they have made and found an important outlet for their experiences and feelings about living with Parkinson's. She also provides telephone support or sends a newsletter to anyone who doesn't want to attend the meetings.

6

Drug treatments

Drugs are the main treatment for Parkinson's and most newly diag-nosed people find that they provide good symptom control. Several different types are available, which may be used on their own or in combination with other drugs. Their aim is to:

- increase the amount of dopamine in the brain (levodopa); or
- stimulate the brain areas where dopamine works (dopamine agonists); or
- block the action of chemicals that reduce the effect of dopamine (these include anticholinergics, entacapone, tolcapone and selegiline); or
- promote the release of dopamine and enable it to stay longer at its site of action (amantadine).

Because each person with Parkinson's is different, the choice of drugs, the doses and the times of day that they are taken have to be tailored to the individual.

The drugs do not stop the progression of Parkinson's, and as the condition develops, they may have to be to be adjusted or new drugs introduced to improve symptom control. Although the drugs are generally very effective, long-term use can lead to side-effects that have to be managed alongside the symptoms of the Parkinson's itself. These side-effects can sometimes be quite disabling. For this reason, some people don't begin drug treatment straight after diag-nosis but wait until their symptoms have developed sufficiently to require medication, concentrating meanwhile on a healthy lifestyle, with a good diet and plenty of exercise and relaxation.

Although there has been some form of medication for Park-inson's since the late nineteenth century, the early treatments were very limited. In the past 30 years there have been enormous advances in the development of anti-Parkinson's drugs. This trend is likely to continue and there is the promise of several new devel-opments in drug treatment within the next few years.

This chapter provides an overview of the drugs currently used in the UK to treat Parkinson's. More information is available from the Parkinson's Disease Society publication *The Drug Treatment of*

Parkinson's Disease (B13), upon which some of the contents this chapter are based.

You will notice that most drugs have two names. One is a generic name, which describes the active ingredient in the medication. The other is a brand or trade name by which the drug is marketed. Both names are given the first time the drug is mentioned with the trade name in brackets and italicized. Thereafter the generic name is used.

Types of drugs

Levodopa

Levodopa is the main drug prescribed to treat Parkinson's and has been in use since the late 1960s.

The aim of levodopa is to increase the levels of dopamine (the neurotransmitter that is in short supply in people with Parkinson's) in the brain. Dopamine cannot be directly replaced because it cannot cross the blood–brain barrier, a barrier that prevents potentially harmful substances in the blood from entering the brain. Levodopa is a chemical compound that can cross this barrier and is then converted into dopamine.

The most commonly prescribed forms of levodopa are co-beneldopa (*Madopar*) and co-careldopa (*Sinemet*). These drugs also contain a substance called a decarboxylase inhibitor, which prevents levodopa from changing into dopamine before it reaches the brain.

For most people with Parkinson's, levodopa can reduce the symptoms of Parkinson's and is considered to be the most effective treatment. The doctor will usually start a patient on a low dose of levodopa, which will be gradually increased until a satisfactory response has been achieved. This process can take some time.

Different preparations of levodopa

Co-careldopa and co-beneldopa are available in a number of different preparations involving different amounts of the drugs they contain.

There are also controlled-release (CR) preparations of both drugs. These release the drug more slowly over a four to six hour period. The benefit of the controlled-release forms is that they can make the effects of the drug last longer because they slow down the absorption of levodopa in the gastrointestinal tract. This may also result in less fluctuation in the levodopa levels in the blood so that the control of symptoms is smoother.

There is also a dispersible form of co-beneldopa, which can be dissolved in water. The benefit of this is that it can be absorbed more quickly than standard versions of levodopa and so starts to work more quickly. It can also be useful for people who have trouble swallowing tablets.

Side-effects

Although co-careldopa and co-beneldopa can be tolerated by most people, some people experience sickness and nausea when they first start taking them. This is usually mild and fades as their body adjusts to the drug.

Although a very effective drug initially, the drawback with levodopa is that with long-term use (usually several years), the body's response to it can become less reliable. The smooth and even control of symptoms that it once produced is no longer dependable, and disabling side-effects can start to occur.

These side-effects can include:

- early wearing off, when the effects of the drug do not seem to last until the next dose is due;
- 'on–off' syndrome, when symptoms can reappear unexpectedly and quickly, which some people describe as being like a light turning on and off, the 'on' period being when the drugs are working and there is good symptom control, and the 'off' period being when the drugs are not working and the Parkinson's symptoms return. This appears to be caused by an interaction between Parkinson's itself and the drug treatment; and
- dyskinesia (involuntary writhing movements), which initially happen when the levodopa level is at its peak, but subsequently may appear at any time.

Management usually involves a change or addition to the drug regimen, such as changing to a controlled-release form of levodopa or adding a drug such as a dopamine agonist to the regimen. Some people who have frequent 'off' periods find that apomorphine (*Apo-go*), a dopamine agonist given by injection, can be beneficial, though it does not help everyone.

Dopamine agonists

Dopamine agonists are a group of drugs that work by stimulating the parts of the brain (know as dopamine receptors) where dopamine works. Unlike levodopa, they don't need to be converted by the brain cells first.

There are two types of dopamine agonists – ergoline and non-ergoline dopamine agonists. These differences relate to the chemical structure of the drugs rather than their action. Ergot is a fungus from which the first dopamine agonist drugs were derived. It has a very distinctive chemical structure, which has been copied in laboratories to make ergoline dopamine agonist drugs. As well as acting on dopamine receptors, ergoline dopamine agonists may also have important effects on other chemical receptors in the brain. There are currently four ergoline dopamine agonists used to treat Parkinson's:

- bromocriptine (*Parlodel*);
- cabergoline (*Cabaser*);
- lisuride (*Revanil*); and
- pergolide (*Celance*).

Non-ergoline dopamine agonists are selective and work on specific dopamine receptors. There are currently three non-ergoline dopamine agonists used to treat Parkinson's:

- apomorphine (*Apo-go*);
- pramipexole (*Mirapexin*); and
- ropinirole (*Requip*).

All of the dopamine agonists are taken orally in tablet or capsule form, apart from apomorphine, which is injected.

Oral dopamine agonists

The oral dopamine agonists are mostly taken several times a day, apart from cabergoline, which is taken once a day because it has a longer duration of action than the others. They are usually introduced slowly, starting with a low dose and gradually increasing the dose until a satisfactory response from the patient's and doctor's viewpoint is achieved.

Some dopamine agonists may be prescribed in the early stages of Parkinson's on their own, but they are commonly used in conjunction with levodopa drugs to improve symptom control in people whose response to levodopa is beginning to vary.

In general, though the degree varies, they have a longer duration of action than levodopa. In recent years, research has shown that dopamine agonists used on their own can be effective in treating Parkinson's for several years and are less likely to cause some of the disabling long-term side-effects associated with levodopa. For this reason, many doctors have tended to start Parkinson's treatment with dopamine agonists, especially in younger people. By using these drugs first, the need for levodopa and the risk of long-term side-effects can be postponed. However, when used alone, dopamine agonists tend to be less effective than the levodopa drugs and some people find that they do not provide enough symptom control.

Side-effects

Dopamine agonists can produce side-effects such as nausea, sickness, confusion, hallucinations and dizziness (from low blood pressure). Some of the ergoline dopamine agonists can also cause rare side-effects, including reddening of the legs and fibrosis of the lungs.

Drowsiness can also be a side-effect of any of the dopamine agonists, but particularly pramipexole and ropinirole. There have been rare cases in the past few years when people taking dopamine agonists have experienced sudden onset of sleep when driving. People who experience this kind of effect should not drive and should discuss the problem with their doctor. However, the UK's Driver and Vehicle Licensing Authority (DVLA) has stated that the risk of sudden onset of sleep is low and that taking Parkinson's drugs should not lead to an automatic cessation of driving.

Apomorphine

Apomorphine is a dopamine agonist that is given either by injection or via a subcutaneous pump. Apomorphine is generally prescribed in addition to other Parkinson's drugs. It is used to treat people who have had Parkinson's for some time, who are finding that their drugs are not working as well as they used to and who are experiencing side-effects such as the 'on–off' syndrome. The people who seem to benefit most are those who have severe 'off' periods but who are reasonably well when they are 'on'.

Apomorphine can be used as a 'rescue treatment' when tablets or capsules fail to take effect. Once injected, it takes between five and 15 minutes to work, which is much quicker than the tablets or capsules. This response is predictable, and as such apomorphine can help some people to go on working for longer than they would otherwise be able to. The drug is also less likely to cause hallucinations and delusions than other Parkinson's drugs (see the section on hallucinations on page 53). For this reason, apomorphine is also commonly prescribed to help people who find that the other Parkinson's drugs do not provide enough balance between mobility and psychiatric side-effects, such as hallucinations, anxiety or delusions.

Side-effects

Because apomorphine can only be given by injection, the person with Parkinson's or the person's carer must be able and willing to give injections. This can provide added restrictions to the lifestyle of a person with Parkinson's. Immobility or rigidity can also sometimes make giving the injection impossible. People with more advanced Parkinson's are sometimes given their apomorphine injections by way of a subcutaneous pump, which they wear and which administers the drug continuously through the course of the day.

Nausea and vomiting are also common problems but these are overcome by giving a drug called domperidone (*Motilium*) before giving the apomorphine injection. Some other drugs used to treat sickness and nausea cannot be given to people with Parkinson's because they make the symptoms of Parkinson's worse (see the sections on drug interactions on page 54 and also the section on drug-induced parkinsonism on page 4) Domperidone is one of the few anti-sickness drugs that doesn't have this effect. Some people also find that they can manage without it after a few months on apomorphine.

Injection sites can become rather sore and irritated, especially with a subcutaneous pump. This soreness can be reduced by diluting the apomorphine with an equal amount of saline (a sterile salt solution). Lumps (nodules) can also occur under the skin – these may disappear with ultrasound treatment. Infection is a potential risk with these lumps, and skin hygiene is very important. If they do become infected, antibiotics are the usual treatment.

COMT inhibitors

COMT inhibitors are a new type of drug used to prolong the duration of action of levodopa. They are used in combination with levodopa drugs. COMT inhibitors block an enzyme called catechol-O-methyl transferase (COMT), which breaks down levodopa. This slows the destruction of levodopa in the body.

Two COMT inhibitors are currently used in the UK to treat Parkinson's:

- entacapone (*Comtess*); and
- tolcapone (*Tasmar*).

Entacapone

Entacapone is taken with each levodopa dose and is generally effective from the start. It particularly helps people who have the 'on–off' syndrome. As well as reducing the 'off' times and increasing the 'on' times, it can often reduce the dose and dosing frequency of levodopa.

A drug (marketed as *Stalevo*) that combines co-careldopa and entacapone has also recently been introduced in the UK. The main benefit is that it is simpler to use because the two drugs have been combined into one.

Tolcapone

Tolcapone is taken three times a day and is also usually effective as soon as the person starts taking it. However, tolcapone has had rather a chequered history as a treatment for Parkinson's in the UK and many other European countries. Soon after it was licensed in 1998, it was withdrawn on the recommendation of the European Medical Agency because there were fears about the liver damage it could cause. After this ruling, the only people in the UK treated with this drug were those whose doctor prescribed it on a named-patient basis. This meant that the doctor took responsibility for using the drug because it was unlicensed. However, in March 2005, following extensive review of prescribing procedures and the information given to the patient, tolcapone was reintroduced in Europe. It can only be prescribed by specialists and anyone treated with the drug has to have regular medical checks and blood tests to check liver function.

Side-effects

COMT inhibitors can increase levodopa side-effects, such as nausea, vomiting and dyskinesia. Where this happens, a reduction in the dose of levodopa taken can often help. Diarrhoea, loose stools and abdominal pain are other possible side-effects. The drug can also cause harmless discoloration of urine which results from ingredients in the drug.

Monoamine oxidase-B inhibitors

Monoamine oxidase-B (MAO-B) inhibitors work by blocking the enzyme monoamine oxidase-B, which breaks down dopamine in the brain. They slow the break-down of levodopa in the brain and are used to make the dose of co-beneldopa or co-careldopa last longer or to reduce the amounts of these drugs that are needed. They can also help to reduce the motor fluctuations that can occur as a side-effect of levodopa.

There are two monoamine oxidase-B inhibitors that are now available to treat Parkinson's:

* selegiline (which comes in two formulations, *Eldepryl* and *Zelapar*); and
* rasagiline (*Azilect*).

These drugs are licensed to be used on their own in early Parkinson's or in combination with levodopa.

Selegiline

Selegiline has been available for some years and is sometimes pre-scribed on its own to treat newly diagnosed people because it may improve the symptoms and delay the need for levodopa. Also, it possibly delays the onset of motor fluctuations.

Over the past few years there has been some conflicting research concerning selegiline. At one time it was thought to slow down the progression of Parkinson's, but then later research suggested that it might increase mortality. Both of these findings are inconclusive.

Selegiline is taken orally either as a tablet (*Eldepryl*) or as an easy-to-take formulation (*Zelapar*) that dissolves quickly on the tongue. Its quick and easy absorption means that a smaller dose is needed to effect control of symptoms.

Side-effects

Selegiline has few side-effects but when taken with co-beneldopa or co-careldopa, the usual side-effects caused by levodopa can occur and may be worsened. If this occurs, the dose of levodopa can be reduced. Selegiline also has a stimulating effect and is usually prescribed as a single dose to be taken in the morning.

Rasagiline

Rasagiline is a new drug that has been licensed from June 2005 as a treatment for Parkinson's in the UK.

Rasagiline is taken once a day. Prescribed on its own in early Parkinson's, it has been shown in clinical trials to provide good symptom control, particularly of tremor and bradykinesia. Research has suggested that, when used with levodopa to treat more advanced Parkinson's, it provides additional therapeutic benefits in people who are experiencing motor fluctuations by reducing 'off' periods and increasing 'on' time without inducing dyskinesia.

Side-effects

Rasagiline seems to be associated with a low incidence of the side-effects (such as hallucinations, oedema, sleepiness and low blood pressure) that can occur with other treatments for Parkinson's.

Anticholinergics

Before the discovery of levodopa, anticholinergics were the only type of drug available to treat Parkinson's. These drugs block the action of acetylcholine, a neurotransmitter that seems to work in balance with dopamine. Because dopamine is in short supply in the brains of people with Parkinson's, this balance is upset. Blocking acetylcholine restores this balance and helps diminish some of the symptoms of Parkinson's.

Anticholinergics are rarely used now, although they are sometimes prescribed on their own to treat younger people in the early stages of Parkinson's who have mild symptoms. They are most effective against tremor. They may also be used to reduce saliva production in people who experience drooling problems and to help people who have a strong, frequent urge to urinate by damping down bladder contractions.

They should not be given to older people because there is an increased risk of confusion. They can also cause dry mouth, constipation and blurring of vision.

Anticholinergics that are used to treat Parkinson's include:

- benzhexol (previously marketed as *Artane*);
- orphenadrine (*Disipal*);
- procyclidine (*Apricolin*, *Kemadrin*); and
- benztropine (*Cogentin*).

Amantadine

Amantadine (*Symmetrel*) is taken orally as a capsule or syrup. It has several functions but is mainly thought to promote dopamine release and allow the neurotransmitter to stay longer at its site of action. Although less commonly used these days, it is occasionally prescribed on its own or in combination with other Parkinson's drugs.

Side-effects

Amantadine has few side-effects and can sometimes help reduce dyskinesia. It also helps some people with tiredness through its stimulatory effect. However, it does not help everyone, and where it does its effects tend to be mild and often short-lived. It can also cause drowsiness, diarrhoea, confusion, swelling of the ankles or a mottled appearance on the skin of the lower leg.

Hallucinations

Some people with Parkinson's experience hallucinations, often visual, occasionally auditory. These are not usually threatening or distressing and in most cases the person understands that they are not real and is able to cope with them. Sometimes, however, they can be frightening.

Hallucinations can affect people with Parkinson's of all ages but are more common in people who have had Parkinson's for a long time and those who are elderly.

They are partly caused by the medication and partly by Parkinson's itself. All the drugs can cause them, but particularly dopamine agonists and anticholinergic drugs. They can also be caused by other conditions such as severely impaired vision, bladder and chest infections, drugs to treat other medical conditions, and dementia. If you do have hallucinations, discuss this with your doctor or Parkinson's disease nurse specialist.

Drug interactions

Many people with Parkinson's are prescribed medication to treat other medical conditions. Many of these medications are quite safe to take with Parkinson's medication, although you should always seek advice from your doctor, Parkinson's disease nurse specialist or pharmacist if you have any concerns.

There are, however, some drugs that can produce Parkinson's symptoms (drug-induced parkinsonism), make existing symptoms worse in people with Parkinson, or cause interactions when taken with Parkinson's medication. These should avoided by people with Parkinson's unless they have been specifically prescribed by a Parkinson's specialist.

Prochlorperazine and metoclopramide

Two of the most commonly prescribed drugs that have this effect are prochlorperazine (*Stemetil*), which is generally prescribed for dizziness, nausea and vomiting, and metoclopramide (*Maxolon*), which is prescribed for nausea and vomiting. Some specialists in care of the elderly say that these two drugs are amongst the commonest causes of parkinsonism in older people.

Some antidepressants

Depression can be common in people with Parkinson's and although many antidepressants are safe to take with Parkinson's medication, there are some that should be avoided. These include:

- fluphenazine with nortriptyline (a combination drug, sold as *Motival* or *Motipress*);
- traylcypromine with trifluoperazine (a combination drug, sold as *Parselin*);
- perphenazine (*Triptafen*); and
- flupenthixol (*Fluanxol, Depixol*).

Calcium channel blockers

Calcium channel blockers, which are drugs that are widely used to treat angina, high blood pressure, abnormal heart rhythm, panic attacks, bipolar disorder (manic depression) and migraine, may also occasionally cause drug-induced parkinsonism. Most of the common agents in clinical practice probably do not have this effect and are likely to be safe to take. The calcium channel blockers that are best documented as causing drug-induced parkinsonism are cinnarizine (*Stugeron*) and flunarizine (*Sibelium*). Do not stop these drugs abruptly but do consult your doctor if you are concerned.

Antipsychotics (neuroleptics)

It is also well-known that a major cause of drug-induced parkinsonism is the antipsychotics (also called neuroleptics), the drugs that are used to treat schizophrenia and other psychotic disorders, such as behaviour disorders in people with dementia. This is because these drugs block the action of dopamine. The longest-established antipsychotics include:

- chlorpromazine (*Largactil*);
- clopenthixol (*Clopixol*);
- haloperidol (*Haldol, Serenace*);
- promazine hydrochloride (*Promazine*);
- supiride (*Domatil, Suparex, Sulpitil*);
- thioridazine (*Melleril*); and
- trifluoperazine (*Stelazine*).

In addition, there are also newer, 'atypical' neuroleptics:

- clozapine (*Clozaril*);
- quietapine (*Seroquel*);
- olanzapine (*Zyprexa*); and
- risperidone (*Risperidal*).

These atypical neuroleptics appear to produce a lower incidence of drug-induced parkinsonism, but they should be avoided by people with Parkinson's unless used by a Parkinson's specialist to treat symptoms such as hallucinations. Olanzapine and risperidone must be used with caution in elderly people with dementia because recent research has suggested that there is an increased risk of stroke if they take these drugs.

Other drugs

Methyldopa (*Aldomet*), used to treat high blood pressure, is also known to sometimes cause drug-induced parkinsonism.

Several other drugs have been reported to cause drug-induced parkinsonism, but as yet there is not enough solid evidence. These include:

- amiodarone, which is used to treat heart problems;
- sodium valproate, which is used to treat epilepsy;
- lithium, which is used to treat bipolar disorder (manic depression); and
- SSRIs (selective serotonin reuptake inhibitors), which are anti-depressant drugs, such as fluoxetine (*Prozac*).

Herbal medicines

Some people are attracted to herbal medicines because they perceive them as a more 'natural' treatment and therefore likely to be better for them than other medications. This is a debatable point. Many drugs are made from plant extracts and even when synthetic, this does not mean that they are inferior to natural products.

The problem with many herbal medicines is that, unlike licensed drugs, they have not been subjected to rigorous scientific research and are not, at present, subject to any government medical control, although regulation is now in progress.

No one with Parkinson's should take any type of herbal medicine without first checking with his or her doctor. Herbal medicines can sometimes contain ingredients that interact with the Parkinson's drugs. An example is St John's wort (hypericum), which is commonly promoted as a treatment for depression. It is known to cause interactions with many prescribed drugs. Some researchers also think that it may be contraindicated for people who have Parkinson's or other movement disorders, but this theory has not yet been substantiated.

Research into new drugs

There have been many advances in the drug treatment of Parkinson's in the past few years, and there is hope of several new developments on the horizon.

All of the current drugs used to treat Parkinson's are given by mouth apart from apomorphine. Alternative drug delivery systems, such as nasal sprays, gels and patches, are an active area of research. Although most studies so far have been inconclusive, a skin patch containing a dopamine agonist called rotigotine has had some positive results in clinical trials. The suggestion is that it may provide 24-hour dopamine stimulation, which would reduce fluctuations and side-effects.

For a long time dopamine was the main focus of drug treatments for Parkinson's. However, research has shown that other systems and substances in the brain may be involved – opioids, glutamate, 5-hydroxytryptamine (5HT, also known as serotonin), adenosine, noradrenaline and cannabinoids. A greater understanding of how these substances are associated with Parkinson's may lead to treatments that work on these systems rather than the dopamine system.

Research into antioxidants (see Chapter 2) may also, in time, lead to the development of new treatments for Parkinson's.

The PD Med Study

The PD Med Study is a large multicentre trial, co-ordinated by the Birmingham Clinical Trials Unit at the University of Birmingham and funded by the NHS Health Technology Assessment programme. The main aim of the study is to assess which class of drugs used to treat Parkinson's provides the most effective control, with the fewest side-effects, for both early-onset and later-onset Parkinson's. The main outcome measures are patient-related quality of life and usage of resources.

Further information is available from the Birmingham Clinical Trials Unit (see Useful addresses).

Talking to your doctor

Don't be afraid to ask your doctor about any of your concerns. He or she cannot help you without knowing what problems you are having, and there are solutions to many difficulties. Remember that, even if the question is embarrassing, you probably won't be the first person who has asked it.

Some people find it helpful to make a list of the things they want to talk about before they see the doctor. Some give it to the doctor when they have their appointment. Keeping a diary can also enable you to keep track of your symptoms, especially if they fluctuate, and help you to describe to your doctor what is happening.

The Patients Association, a voluntary organization that campaigns for patient's rights, publishes a booklet called *You and Your Doctor*, which gives information on how to get the best out of your doctor (see Useful addresses).

There is also a website, <http://www.embarrassingproblems. com>, which includes a section on talking to your doctor (see Useful addresses).

Taking the drugs

As Parkinson's is so individual, don't be surprised if you are taking different drugs from someone else you know who has Parkinson's and don't assume that one treatment is better than another.

Once medication has been prescribed, you will probably need to take it for the rest of your life. Don't stop your medication or change the dose suddenly without first seeking advice from your doctor or Parkinson's disease nurse specialist. When you first start the treatment it might be suggested that you could experiment with the times of the day that you take the medication in order to find the regimen that works best for you. You should, however, keep to the overall daily dose prescribed.

Make sure you have all the information you need to help you make informed decisions about the drugs that have been prescribed for you and that you know who to ask if you have any questions. Your doctor or Parkinson's disease nurse specialist is the best person to advise you.

Personal experiences

Graham

Graham didn't start taking the tablets immediately. He has increased the variety of drugs and amended dosages and timing as his Parkinson's has progressed. 'I feel it is important that I have at least a basic knowledge of the drugs available as I consider the relationship between the specialist and patient as one of partnership. In advance of every meeting I provide him with a resumé of how I see the drug programme, how I have changed since we last met and if I consider that any changes to medication would be appropriate.'

Jeff

Jeff says without the medication he would be incapacitated. He started taking the drugs straight after his diagnosis following a discussion with his specialist. He started on ropinirole and selegiline but now takes levodopa. He sees his neurologist every six months and likes the fact that the doctor asks his opinion and involves him in decisions about his treatment.

Rosemary

Rosemary is on a combination of drugs, the doses of which have been doubled recently because her symptoms had worsened. She takes her medication with her meals to ensure a pattern, otherwise she thinks she would probably forget to take them at the right time. She has a pill box and on Sundays she plans out her medication for the week ahead.

Practicalities

Opening drug packaging, especially blister packs and child-proof bottles, can be a problem for some people if fine movements of the fingers are affected. Your local pharmacist can advise on ways of making this easier, either by dispensing them into easier-to-open containers or, if this is not possible because of the nature of the drug, suggesting gadgets such as bottle openers and foil packet piercers or (if you need to take half a tablet) tablet splitters.

Remembering which medication to take when can also be a

challenge if you are on a complicated regimen. Many people with Parkinson's use special pill boxes and pill timers to help them manage this. Your pharmacist or the Parkinson's Disease Society can advise on what is available.

Hospital admission and your drugs

If you are admitted to hospital, your Parkinson's will be an important consideration for your medical treatment and nursing care – whether Parkinson's or some other, unrelated problem is the reason for your admission. Some people have encountered problems in hospital, especially with regard to self-medicating or getting their drugs at the individual times prescribed for them. If you are going into hospital, discuss this further with your doctor or Parkinson's disease nurse specialist and with the hospital staff before you go.

7

Surgery

Surgical techniques were first used to treat Parkinson's in the 1930s, and until the introduction of the levodopa drugs in the late 1960s surgery was one of the few treatments available. Once levodopa became established, surgery was largely abandoned except to treat people with drug-resistant symptoms.

Although levodopa provided powerful symptom control, over the 10–15 years following its introduction doctors came to realize that it was not a perfect treatment, particularly for people who had had Parkinson's for many years. At the same there were many surgical advances, and developments in computer technology and modern imaging techniques also meant that surgeons were able to pinpoint much more exactly where the surgical target sites were in the brain. A renewed interest in surgery has been the result.

The types of surgery of interest to researchers are:

- deep brain stimulation;
- lesioning (pallidotomy, thalamotomy and subthalamotomy);
- gamma knife surgery;
- neural transplants; and
- infusions of chemicals into the basal ganglia (the part of the brain affected in people with Parkinson's).

Although there have been some promising results, most of these techniques remain experimental.

History of Parkinson's surgery

In the 1930s and 1940s, surgical techniques used involved trying to damage the motor pathways deliberately by making lesions in these parts of the brain. It was hoped by doing this that the symptoms of Parkinson's would be reduced.

The surgery was risky – paralysis was not uncommon – and the results were unpredictable, but advances in the understanding of Parkinson's processes were made as a result of this work.

In the 1950s, the introduction of stereotactic techniques (which

61

enabled three-dimensional targeting of the surgical site) allowed safer and more accurate surgery on the basal ganglia and thalamus (the operations being pallidotomy and thalamotomy), thus avoiding the motor pathways. Lesions could be made in specific areas of the brain that mediate the symptoms of Parkinson's with less risk of paralysis.

Surgery today

Although surgery is a very promising area of research, media stories of miraculous results sometimes promote unrealistic expectations. Surgery cannot cure Parkinson's and it doesn't slow down the progression, but it can provide good symptom control in some people. Most people find that they have to continue to take drugs after surgery, although the dose can often be reduced.

Surgery also carries with it certain risks, and it is generally used only for people who have had Parkinson's for some years and are finding the drug treatment no longer controls their symptoms or for those who have drug-resistant symptoms. Some people are not suitable for surgery – this includes people over the age of 75 and anyone who has confusion, dementia, psychosis, severe depression, cerebrovascular disease or high blood pressure.

Types of surgery

Deep brain stimulation

Deep brain stimulation (also known as Activa Therapy) was pioneered in the 1980s by a research team led by Professors Alim-Louis Benabid and Pierre Pollack in Grenoble, France. The technique is now also performed at several UK centres.

Deep brain stimulation involves the implantation of a wire, with four electrodes at its tip, into one of three target sites in the brain:

- the thalamus – thalamic stimulation, which is used to treat tremor;
- the globus pallidus – pallidal stimulation, which is mainly used to treat people with Parkinson's who have dyskinesia (disabling involuntary movements that are a side-effect of levodopa treatment), although it can also help reduce rigidity and improve 'on' times for people who have the 'on–off' syndrome; and

- the subthalamic nucleus – subthalamic stimulation, which is used to treat tremor, slowness of movement and rigidity, although it can also improve postural stability, gait and freezing; many people who have this kind of deep brain stimulation also find they can reduce their levodopa dose, which in turn reduces the level of dyskinesia and 'off' periods experienced.

Once the wire has been implanted, the surgical team then ensure that the target site has been located accurately. In most centres this is done under local anaesthetic, though in some, general anaesthetic is used. The target site can then be stimulated with a small electric current and the patient's response monitored to confirm that the target localization is accurate. The accuracy of the target localization is confirmed by imaging techniques, such as computed tomography (CT) or magnetic resonance imaging (MRI) (see Chapter 4).

The next step is to connect the wire to a small unit called an implantable pulse generator (IPG). This is planted, under general anaesthetic, under the skin of the chest, rather like a heart pacemaker. The IPG contains the battery and electronics to generate the electrical signals for the stimulation. In the operating theatre the IPG is programmed by the research team with a computer. Once home, the patient can switch this on and off with a hand-held programmer or magnet.

When the stimulator is switched on, electrical signals are sent to the brain to stop or reduce Parkinson's symptoms. When it is switched off, the symptoms return. Deep brain stimulation may be performed on one side of the brain or on both (known as bilateral stimulation). If the stimulation is performed on the right side of the brain, it will affect symptoms on the left side of the body and *vice versa*. Bilateral stimulation only requires one IPG.

Deep brain stimulation has several benefits. Unlike some other forms of surgery, it is non-destructive and reversible. The stimulation can also be adjusted as necessary to ensure the best symptom control possible.

Because deep brain stimulation is a relatively new procedure, the permanency of any positive outcomes achieved and the long-term effects, beyond five to 10 years, are not yet well known.

Side-effects of deep brain stimulation are usually mild, temporary and reversible – they can often be minimized by adjusting the level of stimulation.

People who have had deep brain stimulation should not have diathermy, a treatment using radio frequency energy or sound waves to heat parts of the body. This is performed by a variety of health professionals, usually to reduce muscle and joint swelling and stiffness or to promote tissue healing after surgery or injury. Magnetic resonance imaging (MRI), used in the diagnosis of many other conditions apart from Parkinson's, can also cause problems for people who have had deep brain stimulation, because MRI can produce unsafe heating effects on the implanted electrodes and cause damage. If diathermy or MRI have been suggested to you, ask your Parkinson's doctor or neurosurgeon for advice.

Deep brain stimulation is also being used to treat dystonia, essential tremor and chronic pain, and it has been recently researched as a treatment for depression.

Lesioning

Lesioning involves making selective damage, known as a lesion, to certain cells within specific areas of the brain. As is the case when performing deep brain stimulation, the patient's head is kept in place with the use of a 'stereotactic frame', which is fitted around the head. The target site is located with the aid of computer imaging and then a lesion is made by inserting an electrode with its tip at the optimum point and then passing an electric current through the tip.

There are three main types of lesioning:

- thalamotomy, which targets the thalamus; this is used mainly to treat drug-resistant tremor;
- pallidotomy, which targets the globus pallidus; this is used mainly to treat dyskinesia (which sometimes occurs as a side-effect of the drug treatment), and it can also reduce rigidity and slowness of movement; and
- subthalamotomy, which targets the subthalamic nucleus; this type of lesioning is still experimental and is considered to be a high-risk operation.

Lesioning is not an ideal treatment option because it is irreversible. It is generally performed only on one side because of the high risks associated with two-sided lesioning. However, some bilateral pallidotomies have been performed in order to provide the best symptom control for certain people.

Gamma knife surgery

Gamma knife surgery is a form of radiotherapy. It does not involve any kind of incision, despite its name, but involves directing a source of gamma radiation at the damaged brain tissue through the skull. The effects, when used to treat Parkinson's, are similar to lesioning. This is not considered an acceptable form of surgery for Parkinson's at the moment, because it causes swelling in the brain (oedema) and also because the response of the person with Parkinson's cannot be monitored during the procedure. Therefore it is very rarely used.

Neural transplants

For some years, researchers into Parkinson's have been exploring the possibility of replacing dead and dying dopamine-producing cells with transplanted tissue. The idea is that once the tissue is implanted, the cells in the new tissue will help to raise the dopamine levels in the brain to a more normal level and thereby reduce the symptoms that the person is experiencing. Several different types of tissue have been used for the transplanted material.

Adrenal gland cells are similar to dopamine-producing cells. However, transplant of these cells was abandoned because of the complicated and risky nature of the surgery and because of poor results.

The use of cells from aborted foetuses and embryos was pioneered in Sweden about 20 years ago. In this approach, dopamine-producing tissue is taken from aborted human foetuses at an early stage of development (the foetus is defined as an unborn child after eight weeks' gestation) and transplanted into particular target areas of the brain that are affected by Parkinson's. The hope was that these cells would connect with the rest of the cells in the brain and start producing enough dopamine to stop the symptoms of Parkinson's. Research using embryonic cells was also undertaken (an embryo being defined as an unborn child up to eight weeks' gestation). The results have been very mixed. Although some people improved, mainly those who were under 60 years, others developed adverse side-effects. There are also huge ethical and technical considerations that are not easy to resolve with this type of transplant, such as objections to using aborted tissue and the fact that tissue from several foetuses is needed to obtain enough cells for an effective transplant. This type of implant therefore remains

65

very experimental and is unlikely to become a viable surgical treatment for Parkinson's.

Xenografts involve transplanting tissue from one species to another. Pig foetal dopamine cells have been the focus of Parkinson's xenograft research. The results so far have been largely negative, mainly because the immune system of a person with Parkinson's rejects the implanted cells over time. Research is, however, continuing.

Stem cells are unspecialized cells that have the ability to develop into different types of cells in the body. They are derived from various sources, including the earliest stages of embryo formation (ES cells), the developing nervous system (neural stem cells) and the adult nervous system (neural precursor cells). For the past 10 years approximately, research has looked at whether stem cells could be a source of dopamine cells that might, through transplantation, replace those lost in the brains of people with Parkinson's. Embryonic stem cells are of particular interest because they can develop into most cell types and are easy to isolate. Adult stem cells are not so useful because there are only small numbers of them in the body and they do not reproduce quickly. Although this type of neural transplant offers hope for the future, much more research is needed before scientists will know if this type of therapy has any real potential as a treatment for Parkinson's.

Brain infusions

This type of surgery involves putting a growth factor called glial-derived neurotrophic factor (GDNF) directly into the area of the brain where dopamine is deficient. The hope is that this growth factor will encourage the damaged cells to rejuvenate and produce more dopamine. Initial research was promising but subsequent studies have produced mixed results, and this combined with safety issues have led Amgen, the pharmaceutical company involved, to stop making glial-derived neurotrophic factor. Some researchers dispute this decision and several people in the USA have petitioned Amgen to continue to make it available to those involved in the original trials – so far unsuccessfully.

PD Surg Trial

At present, there is only limited reliable evidence – in the form of randomized controlled trials (the gold standard for medical research into treatments) – as to the best site, technique and timing of surgery for Parkinson's.

The PD Surg Trial is a large multicentre surgical trial, co-ordinated by the Birmingham Clinical Trials Unit at the University of Birmingham, that seeks to:

- evaluate the role of subthalamic and pallidal surgery by either stimulation or lesioning, compared with medical therapy (with surgical intervention delayed for as long as possible) in patients with advanced Parkinson's that is not adequately controlled by their current drug treatment; and
- determine whether early surgery is more effective than deferred surgery for advanced Parkinson's.

Further information is available from the Birmingham Clinical Trials Unit (see Useful addresses).

Personal experiences

Di

Di is 52 and has had Parkinson's for eight years. At the time of her diagnosis she was a busy midwife in a large hospital, having previously worked as a medical ward sister at a teaching hospital and as a senior nurse manager.

Like most people with Parkinson's, she says she had vague symptoms for two to three years before the diagnosis was made. People often commented on her lack of facial expression or told her to 'cheer up'. Her neck tended to be stiff on cold evenings and she found that she was always tripping up when walking. After a while she found that she had difficulties with fine movements of the fingers when carrying out certain tests as a midwife, her shoulder seemed frozen and she often had vertigo, which sometimes resulted in falls.

Her life at the time was demanding and she thought the symptoms might be stress-related. She was juggling a busy career with raising a family, and her husband had just started a new job following redundancy.

One day while on three months' sick leave, she fell in the playground when taking her children to school, and a close friend 'dragged' her to the GP, who admitted her to hospital. She endured a heartrending week where medical opinions on her diagnosis included 'there is nothing neurological wrong with you', 'possibly Parkinson's' and 'motor neurone disease', before the diagnosis of Parkinson's was finally made by a neurologist. To test the diagnosis, he tried her on levodopa–carbidopa, to which she immediately responded. Two months later Di was back at work. Although she was no longer able to deliver babies she continued to use her skills by working in the antenatal clinic for another four years.

Di wanted to keep on working so she was taking quite high doses of levodopa. She found she needed more and more of the drug to keep going, which meant she had a lot of dyskinesia. Five years ago her Parkinson's disease nurse specialist, following discussion with the neurologist, suggested that she might be a suitable candidate for deep brain stimulation. She was petrified at the thought of surgery, as she was one of the first people to have bilateral deep brain stimulation at the hospital where she was treated.

The night before her operation, Di was taken off her medication. This was extremely difficult to cope with and was compounded by the fact that the MRI scanner malfunctioned and she had to be sent to another hospital for the mapping of her head, which helps the surgeon pinpoint the target site for surgery.

The first part of the deep brain stimulation, placing the wires in the head, was done under local anaesthetic, which meant that Di was awake while it was carried out. Prior to this she was fitted with a stereotactic frame under general anaesthetic to keep her head still. She says she doesn't recall anything that was said but she does remember listening to a lot of the Eagles' music – the consultant's favourite at the time. However, she felt her face relax as soon as the surgeon found the spot and inserted the electrode. A week later she had the implantable pulse generator (IPG) connected up to the wires.

In the five years since she had the surgery Di has had a lot of benefit and few side-effects. Although she still takes medication, this has been reduced by a third. Her main problems now are rigidity, dystonia and dyskinesia. She found the deep brain stimulation did help the rigidity. The dystonia disappeared for a while but has recently started to return. She also experiences 'on–offs' about six times a day and manages this with a combination of drugs. Di has noticed that her Parkinson's symptoms tend to return when her general health suffers because of a cold or infection. For some reason at these times her drugs don't seem to work as well. She has regular three-monthly appointments with her Parkinson's disease nurse specialist at the local hospital and also has regular six-monthly appointments with the neurologist at the hospital where she had her surgery.

Di still leads a very active life although she no longer works. In the past year, she has become very actively involved in setting up a Parkinson's Disease Society support group in her local area with her friend Liz, an occupational therapist.

David Beresford

David Beresford is a distinguished South African journalist who writes regularly for UK newspapers such as *The Guardian* and *The Observer*. He has had Parkinson's for over 10 years. He has chronicled his experiences of Parkinson's and deep brain stimulation, which was performed two years ago, in a series of articles for *The Guardian* and in a Channel 4 documentary shown in 2004. He is extremely honest about the effects of his Parkinson's on his life as well as the experience of deep brain stimulation and its after-effects, both good and bad. In a recent piece published in *The Guardian* he said that the operation had produced very positive effects on his tremor and rigidity. However, his speech has worsened, although it is unclear whether this is an effect of the surgery or due to the progression of Parkinson's. You can read his articles on *The Guardian* website – www.guardian.co.uk.

Reading personal experiences or meeting people who have had surgery can help you to understand what is involved and how other people have coped. However, remember that each person is different and that surgery is still quite experimental. As such, there is no guarantee that you would receive the same benefits as other people from surgery.

Further information

Your doctor or Parkinson's disease nurse specialist is the best person to advise you further about surgery and your suitability if you want to be considered. Referral is usually via a Parkinson's specialist.

8

Finances, employment and transport

Depending on your particular circumstances, Parkinson's can have a considerable impact on finances, employment and transport. These are all complicated areas and you should seek expert advice. This chapter considers some of the most common concerns.

Finances

The financial impact of Parkinson's varies. If you are a younger person your concerns might be about earning a living, paying your mortgage, raising your family and saving for a pension. If you are older, you may have paid off your mortgage and no longer be working, but still have worries about how your pension is going to cover the extra costs that most people find they incur as a result of having Parkinson's.

Even if you don't feel you need any financial help at the moment, planning for the future is a good idea.

Welfare benefits and other sources of financial help

Disability benefits are non-means tested and are one of the ways of providing extra income for people with a long-term illness or a disability like Parkinson's. The two disability benefits are Disability Living Allowance (DLA) and Attendance Allowance (AA).

Men and women who are under the age of 65 when they make a first claim may claim DLA. People who are still working can claim it. DLA has two parts:

- a care component that is paid to people who need help with personal care or someone to watch over them to ensure they are safe. There are three rates depending on the amount of care of supervision needed; and
- a mobility component that is paid to people who have difficulty walking out of doors. There are two rates depending on level of need.

AA is for people who make a first claim after the age of 65. There are two rates depending on the amount of help needed with personal care or supervision.

If either of these disability benefits is awarded then extra income may be available through other welfare benefits. Information is available from the Parkinson's Disease Society, the Department for Work and Pensions, Citizens Advice and Age Concern (see Useful addresses) and from local authority welfare rights offices, which should be listed in your telephone directory.

Financial assistance can also sometimes be obtained from other sources, such as trade unions, professional organizations, benevolent funds (such as those tied to the armed services or to particular professions), and national and local charitable trusts. Again, certain organizations can help you to locate these, such as the Disabled Living Foundation, The Directory of Social Change, or Charity Search (see Useful addresses.)

Employment

If you are a young person diagnosed with Parkinson's, one of your prime concerns is likely to be whether you can keep working, and what the alternatives are if you can't. Much depends on what kind of work you do and how your symptoms affect you, but most people find that they can carry on working for several years after diagnosis, provided their symptoms are mild and well controlled by medication. However, some find that as Parkinson's progresses, staying in work can become more difficult and they may need to consider alternative employment or early retirement.

Some personal experiences:

- Karen carried on working for eight years after her diagnosis and was appointed as deputy head for her final three.
- Jeff continues to work as an agricultural worker three years after diagnosis.
- Geraldine Peacock, the former chief executive of Guide Dogs for the Blind, was diagnosed with Parkinson's during a medical examination for the job and went on to run the charity for several years.[29] She now works as a charity commissioner.
- *The Guardian* journalist David Beresford continues to write, 10 years on. His work includes a moving series of articles, pub-

lished in *The Guardian*, about his experiences of living with Parkinson's and of having deep brain stimulation, a surgical treatment for Parkinson's (see Chapter 7). His writing can be viewed on *The Guardian* website (<http://wwwguardian.co.uk).

- Janet Reno worked as the US Attorney General for many years, despite having Parkinson's.

In order to retain as much control over your future as possible, before making any decisions you should obtain as much information and advice about your particular circumstances; your continuing employment; and the options available to you to stay in work, to find alternative work or to retire.

Talking to your current employer should be the first step. Many people find this helps them to accept the fact that they have Parkinson's and to identify future support. Many people whom I interviewed said that their employers and colleagues were sympathetic when they were informed of the diagnosis and often revealed that they had a relative or friend with the condition. In most cases their employers also helped them to find ways to carry on working for as long as possible. For some people, however, telling the employer can be daunting, particularly if they are worried that the response is likely to be unsympathetic or their job may be at risk.

Some employers can be unhelpful and put pressure on the person with Parkinson's to resign or take alternative less well-paid work with the same company. If this is your experience, the Disability Discrimination Act 1995 and 2004 now protects you from discrimination. Since 2004 it has been unlawful for an employer, of any size, to discriminate against disabled people in several areas, including employment.

Your local Jobcentre Plus office should have a Disability Services Team who can advise you on employment options. Financial assistance through the Department for Work and Pensions might also be available to help you meet the costs of travel to work and to purchase equipment that you need to retain or obtain employment.

If you belong to a trade union, staff association or professional body, they should be able to provide you with support and advice.

The Parkinson's Disease Society has an employment pack, which you may find helpful.

Transport

Driving

One of the main concerns most people have when diagnosed is whether they will be able to continue driving. Although Parkinson's can affect driving ability, many people with Parkinson's continue to drive for many years. However, if you hold a driving licence at the time of your diagnosis with Parkinson's you have two legal obligations.

First, you must inform the Driver and Vehicle Licensing Agency (DVLA) in writing that you have Parkinson's. The DVLA will send you a PK1 form (Application for a driving licence/notification of driving licence holder's state of health) to complete and return. In most cases, the DVLA will receive sufficient information from your doctor to issue you with a licence for three years, after which they will review your circumstances. In some cases additional information may be required. This usually involves a driving ability test at a driving assessment centre. However, more than half of those assessed in this way are likely to be given permission to continue driving.

If you have concerns about your driving, you should discuss them with your doctor. The UK also has several specialised driving and mobility centres where you can go for an assessment as well as information and advice about adaptations to make driving easier.

Second, you must tell your insurance company that you have Parkinson's, as failure to do so is likely to invalidate your insurance. Many people are reluctant to tell their insurers about their Parkinson's in case they will be forced to stop driving or end up with increased premiums. This may not be so. If it is, some insurers specialize in insuring disabled drivers and you may be able to obtain insurance from one of these insurers. The Parkinson's Disease Society advisory services can advise further on these companies.

You also have a legal duty to report any later changes in driving ability to the DVLA and your insurance company.

If you are on the higher rate of the mobility component of DLA or if you have a war pension, you may be able to obtain some help from Motability, an independent not-for-profit organisation that provides mobility solutions for disabled people on these benefits (see Useful addresses).

Parking

The Blue Badge scheme is a system of parking concessions designed to help blind people and those with severe mobility problems by allowing them to park close to shops, public buildings and other places. It applies throughout England, Scotland and Wales, with the exception of four central London areas. Application is usually through your local housing or social services office or the town hall. The Blue Badge is automatically awarded to a person who is in receipt of the higher rate mobility component of DLA.

National Key Scheme for disabled toilets

The National Key Scheme for disabled toilets was initiated by RADAR (the Royal Association for Disability and Rehabilitation) in the 1970s. Although it is preferable for all disabled toilets to be kept unlocked, unfortunately many have to be locked to maintain cleanliness and protect them from vandalism and misuse. RADAR's National Key Scheme enables people with disabilities to obtain independent access to over 4,000 locked public toilets around Britain.

To obtain a key you need to write to RADAR (see Useful addresses) with your name and address and a declaration in writing confirming your disability. There is a small charge, which includes packing and postage.

Public transport

If you rely on public transport to get around, there are several initiatives that may help.

The Disability Discrimination Act 1995 gives the government powers to make regulations relating to the design of and access to newly built public transport vehicles such as buses, taxis, coaches, trains and trams. This is to ensure that disabled people can use them.

You may also be entitled to a Disabled Person's Railcard, which entitles you and an accompanying adult to one-third off the price of a rail ticket. Eligibility criteria and application forms are available from main stations or from the Disabled Persons Railcard Office (see Useful addresses).

Local authorities also have discretionary powers to operate concessionary fare schemes for people with disabilities. Such schemes might include a bus or travel pass. For more information on what is available in your area, contact your local authority public transport information office, the details of which should be in the phone book or available from the local Citizens Advice office.

Tripscope, a telephone helpline service offering information and advice on transport issues for people with disabilities, may also be able to advise you further (see Useful addresses).

9

Exercise, sport and leisure

There is no reason why you should not be able to continue exercising, playing sports or doing the activities that you enjoy, although some adaptations may be required. A regular exercise regime and keeping up your interests will help you to cope all the better. This chapter discusses the role of exercise, sport and leisure and highlights some of the many sources of information available.

Exercise

Exercise can have many benefits for people with Parkinson's. Because of the symptoms of Parkinson's, smooth and controlled movement of your muscles and joints can be lost. Mobility, balance and posture are often affected. As well as building up your general fitness and health, a regular exercise regime can help you to overcome some of these difficulties. It also helps you to maintain your abilities, strengthen your muscles and increase the mobility in your joints – all of which in turn help you to remain as independent as possible. Exercise also has enormous psychological benefits, such as alleviating depression, a common feature of Parkinson's.

You need to find an exercise regime that is suitable for your particular circumstances. A physiotherapist can advise you further.

Working with two Sheffield-based physiotherapists, Bhanu Ramaswamy and Richard Webber, the Parkinson's Disease Society has produced *Keeping Moving*, available as a video and booklet (V11) or as a booklet alone (B74). This is an exercise programme that can be used by people with Parkinson's in their homes.[30]

Some people feel more confident about doing exercises in a group. If you are in touch with a physiotherapist, it is worth asking him or her whether there is a class that you can join in your local area. Some local Parkinson's Disease Society branches also run classes.

Karen's branch and Young Parkinson's Support Network (YPSN) group in Leicester have set up a joint exercise class. They felt that some people don't have the confidence to exercise on their own and that access to physiotherapy tended to be at the time of diagnosis or to deal with specific problems. A local private neurophysiotherapist is employed by the branch to run the sessions, which are held in a local council gym. The classes last one and a half hours and include a general exercise and gym programme. Participants include people who are newly diagnosed and those who have had Parkinson's for several years, so there is a mixed range of ability. Exercises are also provided for people to do at home. Karen says that the regular exercise improves her everyday suppleness and she thinks many people benefit from the social contact that the class provides.

Excel 2000 is a charity that helps people to achieve their best potential lifestyle. Their workshops include movement to music, graded to suit each person's level of ability, and information on diet, nutrition and relaxation. Excel 2000 can also provide workshops for people with particular needs or conditions, including for those with Parkinson's and their carers, as well as video and audio tapes for people to use at home (see Useful addresses).

Sport and leisure

Sport and leisure activities keep you mentally alert as well as reducing or preventing depression, stress and boredom. Many of the people I interviewed said their sport or leisure activities helped to improve their confidence and stopped them becoming obsessed by Parkinson's. They also stressed the importance of the social interaction and friendships these activities provided.

Personal experiences

Jonathan

Jonathan loves sports, particularly cycling, swimming and skiing. In fact he noticed his first symptoms while exercising. When he was cycling he noticed that his heel kept hitting the cycle frame as he pedalled and when he was swimming he noticed that the acceleration was lacking when he kicked his legs. Since diagnosis he has had to make some adjustments but remains a keen sportsman. He still cycles to the shops daily but doesn't go for the long rides he used to. Jonathan also has an exercise bike and cycles four miles on this every day. He would like to start swimming again but finds it difficult to co-ordinate both arms and legs. He hopes to go skiing again if he can find someone to go with him to act as a 'buddy' to give him confidence.

Anne

When Anne was diagnosed with Parkinson's she was determined not to just sit in a chair but to continue with her hobbies. She loves badminton and still plays regularly with an over-50s club. Dancing too has always been a big part of her life. When tap dancing became impossible because of her Parkinson's, she took up line dancing.

Whatever sport you are interested in, there is likely to be an organization to advise you further. Loss of confidence can often be a stumbling block, but some of the sporting organisations for people with disabilities have 'buddy' or similar schemes, which enable you to enjoy your favourite sport in the company of others.

Gardening

We are a nation of gardeners in the UK, whether this involves a few indoor pot plants, window boxes or a full-scale garden. If this describes you, there is no reason to stop gardening just because you have Parkinson's, even if you need to make some adjustments. As well as providing you with fresh air and exercise, it will give you a creative outlet.

An occupational therapist can advise you on ways of overcoming particular problems you have with gardening, including advice on tools. There are also organizations that specialize in gardening and horticultural therapy such as Thrive and Gardening for the Disabled Trust (see Useful addresses).

Personal experience

For Susan, life is all about gardening. Living as she does in an idyllic rural spot, she often spends the first moments of the day with a cup of coffee in one hand pottering about in her garden. Although her Parkinson's makes some tasks more difficult, she says nothing will stop her from gardening. She tends to use plastic rather than terracotta pots because they are lighter to carry. Planting with seeds is now impossible because she can't manage the fine movements of the fingers that are necessary. Instead she buys plug plants, which are easier for her fingers to manage. Gardeners traditionally like to share information and ideas. Her many friends in her local garden club are always willing to help her with any tasks she can't manage in return for a cup of tea, a slice of cake and cuttings from her garden!

As well as developing your own garden, you may also be interested in visiting gardens and stately homes. Many organizations, such as English Heritage, the National Trust and the National Gardens Scheme, can provide accessibility guides or information about facilities for people with disabilities.

Creative arts

Creative activities, such as music, art and writing, seem to be particularly popular among people with Parkinson's. As well as the creative enjoyment they provide, they can also give you a valuable outlet for expressing your feelings.

The following professional creative artists have been interviewed for the Parkinson's Disease Society membership magazine, *The Parkinson*. Three of them have Parkinson's and one is a carer.

Personal experiences

Rosalind Grimshaw

Rosalind Grimshaw, an internationally renowned stained glass artist, was diagnosed with Parkinson's in 1984 at the age of 37. Since then she has continued to work professionally and has recently completed a large-scale commission – a 'Creation Window' for Chester Cathedral. This stunning window depicts the six days of creation and includes a scan of Rosalind's brain showing the depletion of dopamine. *Six Days*, a beautifully illustrated book written by her friend, Painton Cowan, tells the story of the window and quotes Rosalind and her partner, Patrick Costeloe, on living with Parkinson's. Rosalind says that she refuses to allow her Parkinson's to stop her from working and feels that it has paradoxically brought about an intensely creative period in her life.

Barbara Thompson

Barbara Thompson is a well-known jazz saxophonist and composer, diagnosed with Parkinson's in 1994. Barbara continued her career as a professional musician for several years, including a 50-date 'Thompson's Tangos' concert tour with her band Paraphernalia. Although Barbara has retired from performing professionally, she still plays for pleasure. She is now a full-time composer and in 2003 premiered a choral piece 'Journey to an Unknown Destination', commissioned by Norwich Arts.[31]

Charlotte Johnson Wahl

Charlotte Johnson Wahl is a professional artist based in London, who was diagnosed with Parkinson's in 1989. She specializes in oil landscapes and portraits. These days her paintings tend to focus on interiors of her flat, views from the window or people who visit her. Breaking through the listlessness that the Parkinson's causes can be challenging but she says it is worth it.[32]

Nancy Tingey

Nancy Tingey is an artist, art curator and teacher, whose husband Bob has had Parkinson's for many years. Nancy has been running 'Art with Parkinson's' groups since 1994, first in Australia and now in the UK.[33, 34] Participants use materials that are easy to hold and immediately rewarding to use, such as good-quality oil pastels and wet-on-wet water-colours. People with Parkinson's benefit from increased self-confidence and self-esteem, a sense of achievement, improved quality of life – and often a reduction in symptoms when the creative activity takes over. (See Useful addresses for the Art for Parkinson's website.)

Computers

Many people have found that having a computer has made an enormous difference to their lives, not only helping them with day-to-day business and letters, but also helping them to keep in touch with others and obtain information about Parkinson's from the internet. On-line shopping and banking can also make a lot of difference to people who have problems with mobility.

Occupational therapists can advise about getting a computer or an electronic typewriter and about any funding available. There is also a specialist voluntary organization called AbilityNet, which aims to make computer technology accessible to people who have disabilities (see Useful addresses).

Computer courses may also be run by colleges and adult education facilities in your local area. Further details can be obtained from your local library or your local authority education office. UK Online is a government initiative that aims to provide internet facilities. Learndirect also offers computer courses that can be studied at home if you have internet access or at a local learndirect centre (see Useful addresses).

Personal experience

Gerry is in his early 40s and has had Parkinson's for seven years. He didn't know anything about computers until one of his friends suggested he did a course at the local college. He now does everything on the computer, not just for himself, but for his local YPSN group, his Parkinson's Disease Society branch and his church.

Gerry says that being able to buy on-line has revolutionised his life. He says he compares the price of everything on-line before he buys it – going around several shops to do the same would be impossible for him.

One of the greatest pleasures is communicating with other people with Parkinson's. The internet is wonderful for people like Gerry who often can't sleep, or for those who find getting out of the house difficult. Gerry says that it brings the world into the front room and lessens the isolation that many people with Parkinson's feel, especially those living in rural areas. Gerry also uses the computer to keep up to date with developments in Parkinson's research.

Holidays

There is no reason why having Parkinson's should stop you from enjoying your holidays as much as you have always done. Careful planning helps.

The Parkinson's Disease Society publishes an annual *Holidays and Respite Care Guide*, which contains information on short stays, respite care and holidays for people with Parkinson's and their carers and families.

The Calvert Trust (see Useful addresses) specializes in providing outdoor activities, such as sailing, rafting, climbing, abseiling, archery, horse riding and swimming, for disabled people, with skilled staff.

Ian, a Parkinson's Disease Society area officer, has organized activity breaks with the Trust. He says, 'The benefits of such breaks to people with Parkinson's are numerous. Because the emphasis is on what people can still achieve rather than what is no longer possible, the confidence of participants grows, new friendships are made and many people leave with the desire and incentive to continue with exercise and activities when they return home.'

Holiday Care is an organization that advises people with disabilities and special needs about holidays (see Useful addresses).

Travelling abroad[35]

Again, the secret is to plan carefully before you go. Book with the airline well in advance of your travel date and make sure you tell them about any special assistance you require.

It is very important to take a letter from your doctor stating that you have Parkinson's disease and that you are fit to travel. The letter should also give details of the medication that you have been prescribed. This will help you if there are any queries about your medication at customs or you run into any difficulties while you are abroad.

Taking medicines abroad is another issue. Although you should be able to take as much of your prescription medicines as you need, some countries require you to obtain an import permit to bring in some types of prescribed drugs for personal use – check with the embassy of the country to which you are travelling.

Make sure your medication is in your hand luggage and take extra supplies with you just in case your medication is not available in the country you are visiting.

Check what the health service arrangements are for the country you are visiting (see the travel advice section of the Department of Health's website, www.doh.gov.uk). You should also ensure that you have adequate insurance, and, if travelling to a European Union (EU) country make sure you apply for a European Health Insurance card (EHIC) (available from your local post office) and take it with you.

10

Emotional and psychological impact

Parkinson's can have significant emotional and psychological effects and these can be the most difficult aspects of learning to live with the condition. How these will affect your life will depend on many factors – your personality, your attitude to life, your circumstances and the support available to you.

How you react to the diagnosis will be governed to a large extent by two factors – your expectations of the condition, and the knowledge that you already have of Parkinson's. A realistic outlook is important, but don't be surprised if this takes you some time. It is not uncommon for people to have extreme reactions while they are coming to terms with the diagnosis. Some automatically assume that they will become very disabled and have to give up everything they love in life to take on an 'invalid's' role. Others deny that there is anything wrong with them and try to cope without any help, even when they have considerable difficulties. Your ideas may also be based on a relative who had Parkinson's many years ago. Remember that developments in the understanding and treatment of Parkinson's are being made all the time, and your experience may be very different.

Most of the people I interviewed said that their self-esteem and confidence had been affected by Parkinson's. They also talked about how their sense of identity and other people's perceptions of them were thrown into question by having the condition. Many had to redefine these as a result, especially if having the condition led to changes in their life. Although this was understandably often a difficult process, some people experienced positive outcomes and enjoyed new, satisfying challenges.

Michael J. Fox's story, told candidly in his autobiography *Lucky Man*, provides a good example of this. He describes his responses to having Parkinson's, which began with denial before eventually moving on to acceptance. He also describes his Parkinson's as being 'a gift', despite the disability that he experiences.

Acknowledging your feelings and finding help

However difficult it is for you, try to acknowledge and accept your feelings, whatever they are. If you feel overwhelmed, try to find someone to talk to about them. This might be a partner, a relative or friend – someone who knows you well and with whom you feel comfortable.

For some people, however, discussing their feelings with someone who is not closely involved in their life can be easier, especially if they don't want to upset someone close or are afraid of the reaction that person might have. Many people find talking things over with someone else with Parkinson's or with another carer through a local Parkinson's Disease Society branch or YPSN (Younger Parkinson's Support Network, formerly YAPP&Rs) can be very helpful. If you don't want to meet people face to face or if you live in an area with no support group nearby, there are also several discussion forums on the internet (see Useful addresses).

Discussing your feelings with a health or social care professional is another approach. This might be a Parkinson's disease nurse specialist, a member of the Parkinson's Disease Society advisory line staff or a local community support worker. You might also find it helpful to talk to a professional counsellor. Counselling involves using psychological or talking therapies to help you to look at your life and the feelings you have in a safe environment. It is not about giving advice but providing space and time to you to help you to explore your feelings and behaviour to gain insight into what you find most difficult and why. This can help you to resolve your feelings, accept your situation or make changes to your life.

Finding a creative outlet, such as writing, art or music, for your feelings and experiences can also be beneficial. Coping with the emotional and psychological aspects of Parkinson's can also be helped by two important factors – attitude and access to reliable information about Parkinson's and related subjects. Both these subjects are discussed in Chapter 11.

Relationships

Relationships of all kinds – intimate, platonic, private and professional – can be affected by Parkinson's. The communication problems that the condition causes can make starting or joining in conversations harder. The lack of facial expression or body language can paint a misleading picture of the person to other people and result in misunderstandings. People with Parkinson's may appear uninterested or hostile when they are not, and intimate gestures that were part of a couple's unspoken language – smiling at each other or squeezing a hand – may become more difficult for the person with Parkinson's to do.

Some reversal of roles can also take place. For instance, the carer may have to take on more of the domestic chores than previously. The person with Parkinson's may have to give up work and the carer may become the main breadwinner. Losing life roles can make the person with Parkinson's feel bereaved, powerless and lacking in self-esteem. The carer on the other hand can feel that he or she has too many responsibilities and can therefore feel very stressed. All of this can lead to resentment and tension, feelings that may be exacerbated if there are worries about the future, or financial concerns.

The psychological and emotional impact can also make some people reluctant to engage in social activities and become introverted. This may be partly caused by the loss of self-esteem and communication problems discussed earlier. Tiredness can also be a factor. Some people also feel embarrassed by their symptoms, especially if someone they know has been unsympathetic. The loss of social status because of changes in their life, such as giving up work or role reversals within their personal life, can also contribute to this. The effect may also be to make the person's family isolated.

Sexual relationships

Although Parkinson's can affect sexual relationships, it is important to stress that this doesn't mean you will have problems. We live in a very sexualized world and it is easy to lose sight of the fact that the sexual and intimate needs of each person and each couple are different. For some, a happy intimate life is having sex often, whereas others are quite content if they make love once or twice a month or show intimacy through hugging and kissing. It only becomes a problem if you or your partner becomes unhappy with the nature of your sexual and intimate life or how it is expressed. If this is the case, then help and advice are available.

You may find that Parkinson's does restrict what you can do

physically and when you can do it. If this is the case, you may need to adapt to circumstances! For example, although you may have previously found that the evenings were the best time for making love, your Parkinson's may mean that this is not now your best time – if so, find a time when your medication is working well when being intimate is easier.

Fatigue, stress and depression can be common in both the person with Parkinson's and the carer. Both parties can get so caught up in managing Parkinson's that they find it hard to switch off from this to concentrate on their intimate relationship. As discussed in the previous section, changes in communication ability can also cause misunderstandings.

Often the answer lies in talking about these things with your partner. Help and support are also available from professionals, such as psychosexual counsellors. If you feel too shy or find it too hard to verbalize your concerns, try giving your doctor or Parkinson's nurse specialist a written list of questions. The Parkinson's Disease Society advisory line nurses may also be able to help.

Sometimes the symptoms of Parkinson's and the side-effects of the drugs can cause physical problems, such as erectile dysfunction or increased libido and, very occasionally, behavioural problems. If these occur, you should discuss them further with your doctor or Parkinson's nurse specialist.

Spirituality

Being diagnosed with a chronic health condition like Parkinson's can have a profound effect on your spirituality.

Spirituality can be defined in many ways. For some, it is a religious faith that defines who they are as a person and that influences everything they do in life as well as their attitudes and feelings. For others, it is more about their sense of self and the things that matter to them or their outlook on life. This will involve different things for different people – what they do for a living, their family, the music they like or the football team they support, creative activities, their garden and so on.

For some people the effects are positive. Having Parkinson's enriches their spiritual life and makes them realize what is really important in their life. Any religious or spiritual experience that they already have becomes deeper and leads them to explore issues that they had never previously considered. Churches, synagogues, temples, mosques and community cultural centres can provide tremendous support.

For other people, the consequences can be more unsettling. Having Parkinson's can make them question everything that they believed in. If they have a religious faith, the diagnosis of Parkinson's can make them feel abandoned by the God from whom they previously obtained a lot of comfort and strength. Others, who are not religious, may find that Parkinson's threatens something that made up a large part of their sense of self, such as a chosen career from which they derived enormous satisfaction. This may lead to a spiritual crisis. People who have had to give up something because they have Parkinson's say that finding alternatives to replace what they had to give up helped them to deal with the feelings of loss that they felt.

Because spirituality is so individual, there are no simple answers to managing the impact that Parkinson's may have on yours. There is also very little about it in the literature on Parkinson's. Finding someone to talk to about how you are feeling may be the first step, whether a friend or family member, someone through your place of worship, a chaplain at your local hospital or a professional counsellor.

You may find some of the resources and ideas mentioned in Chapter 11 useful. The *Parkinson's Disease Self-Care Manual*, published by Foundation September, a Dutch medical publishing company, in association with the NHS Executive, has a chapter on 'Spiritual Welfare', written by the Revd Dr P. Bellamy, which explores the nature of spirituality, how it is expressed, how spirituality is affected by a diagnosis of Parkinson's, living with the illness, and finding supportive networks. See Foundation September's website for more information on obtaining this resource, <http://www.parkinsonsupdate.org>.

You may also have a religious faith or be from a culture that means that you have particular attitudes or requirements regarding certain medical treatments or procedures. For instance, dietary factors might also be an important consideration if you have to go into hospital or for respite care. If you do have these sorts of concerns, discuss them with your doctor, Parkinson's disease nurse specialist or the other health or social care professionals who are involved in your care.

Depression

Depression and mood problems are common features of Parkinson's. Depression is more than the feelings of sadness and being fed up that we all experience from time to time. These usually don't last very long and have minimal impact on our daily lives. Depression is a recognized illness that is described by the Depression Alliance as an 'intense feeling of persistent sadness, helplessness and hopelessness accompanied by physical effects such as sleeplessness, a loss of energy, or physical aches and pains'.[36] Depression in people with Parkinson's is complicated. Biological changes in the brain may be partly responsible. Dopamine, the substance that is decreased in the brains of people with Parkinson's, is one of three neurotransmitters involved in depression, and research suggests that the others, serotonin and noradrenaline, may also have some links to Parkinson's. As well as this, however, depression in many cases will also be a response to the psychological and emotional impact of having Parkinson's.

Although depression can occur at any time, there are certain stages of Parkinson's and certain times in a person's life when depression is more likely.

Obviously, the time of diagnosis can be particularly difficult. In due course, people often adapt to Parkinson's, particularly if they have a good response to drugs and other treatments, but may then experience depression if the condition progresses and symptoms become more pronounced. Any times involving change or stress, such as giving up work or activities, can also make people more vulnerable to depression.

Diagnosing depression can be difficult in Parkinson's. This is because some of the symptoms of Parkinson's can also be features of depression, such as fatigue, sleeplessness, the stooped posture, a quiet monotonous voice and difficulties with facial expression. As a result, some people may be mistakenly diagnosed as depressed when they are not, while depression in others may go undiagnosed.

The symptoms of Parkinson's alone don't seem to be the most important determinant in what makes certain people depressed. Someone who is very depressed may only have mild symptoms of Parkinson's – whereas someone with severe symptoms of Parkinson's may not experience depression at all. Depression can also be common in carers, particularly if they have to take on a lot of responsibilities.

If you are experiencing symptoms of depression, it is important that you seek advice from your doctor. You may need your Parkinson's medication adjusted, or the doctor may prescribe anti-depressants. These can work very well but some are more suitable for people with Parkinson's than others (see Chapter 6).

Counselling or other psychological treatments may also help, as may joining support groups, either through the Parkinson's Disease Society or through another organization (see Useful addresses).

Regular exercise and relaxation are also important in dealing with depression (see Chapter 9).

Cognitive problems

Although the intellect is unaffected in many people with Parkinson's, some do experience problems, either as a result of the biological impact of the condition or from side-effects of medication.

Some people have problems with remembering, or concentrating for very long. Slowness of thinking can also be a feature. Many people find they need extra time to respond to someone who is talking to them. It is not that they don't understand what is being said to them, it just takes them longer to process their thoughts and formulate answers to questions they are asked. Doing more than one thing at once can be difficult.

About 15–20 per cent of people with Parkinson's do develop dementia, and this is more common in people with late-onset Parkinson's disease and in people in whom the condition progresses more rapidly.[37] Some other forms of parkinsonism, such as dementia with Lewy bodies, have dementia as a predominant feature. Some people, particularly those who are older, may have coexisting conditions that cause cognitive problems or dementia (see Chapter 13).

Some of the drugs used to treat Parkinson's can also cause psychiatric side-effects such as hallucinations (see Chapter 6). Treatment of all these factors can be complicated and it is important to discuss any cognitive problems you may experience with your doctor.

For anyone who wants to read more about any of the issues discussed in this chapter, I recommend *Parkinson's Disease: a Self-Help Guide* by Marjan Jahanshahi and C. David Marsden.

11

Self-help

Self-help plays an important role in the management of Parkinson's but, as with everything else about Parkinson's, there is no one standard prescription. You have to find an approach that works for you. This may mean adjusting your attitude or educating yourself about Parkinson's, trying complementary therapies, or meeting others in a similar position. Helping others can also be a great motivator – through raising awareness of Parkinson's, fund-raising, being involved in running a support group or developing a resource such as a website or book based on your experiences. This chapter explores some of the different ways you can help yourself to cope with Parkinson's.

Attitude

No one is going to pretend that having Parkinson's is always easy, although most people say keeping positive is the secret to coping.

Svend Andersen was diagnosed with Parkinson's in 1989 at the age of 39. He is a Danish clinical psychologist who works part-time. He is also a founder member of the DANYAPPERS, a Danish group for younger people with Parkinson's and their families, and a board member of the European Parkinson's Disease Association.

Svend has explored the issue of how best to cope psychologically when you have a chronic condition such as Parkinson's. His ideas have been presented at European Parkinson's Disease Association conferences and published as a Parkinson's Disease Society information sheet, *The New Role of the Patient* (FS16) and in a book, *Health is Between Your Ears: Living with a chronic disease*, which many people with Parkinson's find inspiring (see Further reading).

'I remember', he writes in an editorial in *Focus*, the magazine of the European Parkinson's Disease Association,[38] 'the EPDA's first international young onset conference in Peterborough, UK, in 1994. The title of the conference was: "To hell with Parkinson's".

'Normally when people are diagnosed with Parkinson's, they – without thinking about it – move into a culturally created role. At this conference I met some of the most 'crazy' people with Parkinson's; they did not want to be restricted by a culturally defined role. They had, in spite of Parkinson's, a high quality of life; they encompassed themselves and their disease with acceptance and love. They had humour, courage and were active in many ways.

'For me this conference was a turning point about being a patient and the patient's role. It is troublesome to live with Parkinson's, but it is at the same time possible to live a good life. It was an experience that demonstrated to me that quality of life is not about the severity of the disease, but about how you choose to relate to life, yourself and your disease. And when the disease closes some doors, it is important not to use all your energy looking at the closed door, otherwise you will not see all the new doors that open.'

The Expert Patients Programme

The Expert Patients Programme is the government's NHS-based training initiative, which also recognizes the importance of patient empowerment.

A definition of 'expert patients' is 'people living with a long-term health condition, who are able to take more control over their health by understanding and managing their conditions, leading to an improved quality of life'.

The programme is based on research from the UK and USA over the past 20 years that shows that people living with chronic illnesses are often in the best position to know what they need to manage the condition they have. If they are given the necessary self-management skills, they can make a considerable impact on the management of their condition and their quality of life, feeling more confident and in control.

To become an 'expert patient' you take a six-week course lasting two and a half hours each week, which is led by someone who lives with a long-term in condition.

Karen first joined this scheme as a participant but subsequently felt that she could use her teaching skills to good effect by becoming a tutor. She finds the experience different from classroom work. She says she always feels a bit nervous before she tutors on this programme because her confidence has been affected by having Parkinson's. However, she does enjoy meeting people with other chronic conditions as well as those with Parkinson's.

More information can be obtained from the Expert Patients Programme enquiry line or website (see Useful addresses.)

Finding information

The amount of information that people want about Parkinson's and related subjects varies enormously. Some people want the facts but don't want to delve too deeply, preferring to live each day as it comes and asking for information when something crops up that they need help with. Others are hungry for information, wanting to know as much as possible so they can be prepared and make plans accordingly. You have to decide what works best for you.

Resources on Parkinson's

The first place to start in the UK if you want more information on Parkinson's is the Parkinson's Disease Society, which is a voluntary organization that supports people with Parkinson's, their families and professionals who are involved in their care. The Society's activities include promoting and funding research into Parkinson's, campaigning and raising awareness, and developing resources and projects to help anyone affected by Parkinson's.

The Parkinson's Disease Society has a wide variety of booklets and information sheets on Parkinson's and related subjects, as well as regional networks, which provide help on a more local level (see Useful addresses).

The European Parkinson's Disease Association also has a wealth of information on their website (<http://www.epda.eu.com>), including personal accounts and links to other sites (see Useful addresses).

Medical information and the media

Developments in information technology, such as the internet, have made an enormous quantity of information more easily accessible. Although there are some excellent sites, there are also many that contain inaccurate or dubious material, particularly in the field of complementary therapies, which attracts many genuine practitioners but also a lot of people peddling all sorts of 'miracle cures'. Many of these are marketed in a way that makes them seem more credible than they are, often making claims that 'research has proved their efficacy'.

A study by Dr Katja Schmidt and Professor Edzard Ernst at the Peninsula Medical School of the Universities of Exeter and Plymouth demonstrates how faulty some of the advice and claims made for some products can be. These authors analysed 32 popular websites that give advice and information on various complementary therapies used to treat cancer and found that a significant number of these were a risk to people with cancer. However, two sources of excellent information on complementary therapy research were identified – *Bandolier* and Quackwatch (see Useful addresses).

The British Medical Association (BMA) publishes a guide, 'Finding reliable health information on the internet', on its website, <http://www.bma.org.uk>.

DISCERN is a questionnaire that looks at how to assess written information on treatment for a health problem. The project is based at the Division of Public Health and Primary Health Care, Institute of Health Sciences, University of Oxford. See the website, <http://www.discern.org.uk>, for more information.

The National Electronic Library for Health (NeLH) is a digital library being developed in the UK to provide reliable information to help people make decisions about their health. This includes a 'Hitting the Headlines' section, which analyses media stories and how reliable they may be (see <http://www.nelh.nhs.uk>).

If you are particularly interested in research, the Parkinson's Disease Society has a group called SPRING (Special Parkinson's Research Interest Group), which looks at the latest developments and findings (see Useful addresses).

Complementary therapies

Complementary therapies are particularly popular among people who have long-term conditions, such as Parkinson's. Examples include acupuncture, the Alexander technique, aromatherapy, ayurveda, creative therapies (involving art, music, dance or drama), chiropractic, conductive education, herbal medicine, homoeopathy, osteopathy, Pilates, reflexology, tai chi and yoga.

While conventional medicine can provide good symptom relief, it does not always provide all the answers. Most people want to do all they can to help themselves and see complementary therapies as a possible answer. Sometimes people become disillusioned with mainstream medicine, while others are simply reluctant to take drugs.

Complementary therapies also tend to use a holistic approach, that is, one that treats patients as a whole, not only treating the disease but also taking into account the person's physical and mental state as well as his or her social background.

The division between orthodox medicine and complementary therapies has become more blurred over the past few years. Some complementary therapies now have well-established uses in mainstream medicine, such as acupuncture for pain relief and creative therapies for people with mental health problems. Some conventional health practitioners may also train in complementary therapy techniques. The term 'integrated medicine' is increasingly used to cover this approach, though some conventional doctors still have reservations about complementary therapies.

Complementary therapies should always be used in addition to conventional medicine, not instead of it. If you are thinking of trying complementary therapies, discuss this further with your doctor or Parkinson's disease nurse specialist first. Make sure the complementary therapist you use is properly trained and affiliated to a recognized regulating professional body for the complementary therapy discipline in question.

Around a year after his diagnosis, Chris took part in a trial of the Alexander technique in relation to Parkinson's.[39] 'This was very useful, although because I was still only in the early stages, some of the teachings went over my head because I hadn't seen or experienced some of the symptoms the particular movements were designed to help with.' Chris also learnt transcendental meditation some years ago, and uses some of the tips and techniques of both complementary therapies to help him in everyday life. For instance, when off-balance, he remembers that the Alexander technique teacher taught him to look over people's heads to help offset this.

Living alone

Living with Parkinson's can seem more daunting if you live alone. This can be compounded by assumptions made by many health professionals and much of the literature available that there will be a carer involved. Yet many people do live alone with Parkinson's, either through choice or circumstance, and many of them manage very well as long as they have the help they need to overcome any particular problems.

As well as providing support through local branches, the Parkinson's Disease Society and Help the Aged have information sheets on living alone, which cover many of practical issues, such as security, safety and emergencies (see Useful addresses).

Personal experience

Jonathan is 55 and lives on his own in Suffolk. Three years ago he was diagnosed with akinetic–rigid syndrome (see Chapter 1). Jonathan has always led an active life. He worked in research and development at British Telecom for 37 years until he retired in 2004. He has a busy social life and a keen interest in sports, particularly skiing, cycling and swimming. His girlfriend lives in Germany and they commute between their two countries on a regular basis to see each other.

Jonathan's main problems are with rigidity, mobility and balance, constipation, and fatigue. Jonathan says that his reaction at first was to remain detached from the process of being diagnosed and treated. He saw it as a mechanical series of events – a problem that needed to be dealt with.

Most of his colleagues knew he had the condition. Some were quite moved by the news and were very supportive. Jonathan was encouraged by the fact that one of his colleagues knew someone who had had Parkinson's for 20 years who was still active and able to drive. However, although Jonathan carried on working for some time after his diagnosis, he eventually decided to take voluntary redundancy when it was offered because he felt he wasn't performing his work properly. One of his colleagues was also very difficult, making Jonathan's working life stressful, and this also spurred him on to make a change in his life. Leaving work was hard and he might have stayed if more flexible working and support could have been arranged. He doesn't think that his employers really understood the needs of people with progressive illnesses or the need for flexible working. The emphasis was on performance – as a result he was offered a course on maximizing his performance but no support to help him perform.

Jonathan is used to living on his own and, although some things present problems, he manages his day-to-day activities himself. He wants to remain as independent as possible. There have been some changes in his routine, such as employing a cleaner once a week. Fine movements of the fingers, as in ironing and managing buttons, are particularly difficult for him, so shirts, which he used to like wearing, are proving to be too hard to manage. Making model engines, a favourite hobby, is also proving harder but he maintains his interest by writing historical and 'how to' articles for specialist model-making magazines.

Jonathan still drives, though he switched to an automatic car, which he finds easier to manage, and he still cycles around town. Jonathan feels frustrated by the fact that he is not disabled enough for some benefits that would make his life easier, like a blue badge for parking and a disabled person's railcard. He would like to employ someone to iron his shirts but is unable to afford to do so on his pension. There are several health and disability support groups in his area and, even though he is reluctant to ask for help, knowing they are there if he needs them gives him confidence in coping with his everyday life.

His greatest support comes from his girlfriend and his many friends. He found telling them a difficult and upsetting experience because he felt they perceived him as a fit person. However, one of his friends has a mother with Parkinson's so knows exactly what Jonathan is dealing with.

He is also a member of his local Parkinson's Disease Society support group. He says he was reluctant to go at first because he was worried that he would see people much worse than himself. In fact he has found it very supportive and enjoys sharing tips on coping with symptoms.

Finding your own way

Sometimes people use their own life experiences and interests to find their own methods of self-help and helping other people. Karen, who is profiled in Chapter 12, used her experiences as teacher to develop a book for young children on Parkinson's. Svend, the psychologist mentioned earlier in this chapter, focused on how best to cope psychologically with having a chronic condition such as Parkinson's. Michael J. Fox used his celebrity to set up

a foundation to promote Parkinson's research. You may also dis-
cover your own unique way of helping yourself that turns out to
also be of value to other people with Parkinson's.

Personal experience

Chris lives in London with his partner and was diagnosed with
Parkinson's in 1997 at the age of 37 after having symptoms for
about two years. He has used a variety of creative ways to help
himself.

Chris is employed full-time doing sales analysis for British
Telecom and has negotiated with them to work at home. He is sure
that stress plays a big part in his Parkinson's and he has noticed
that his symptoms really accelerated a few years ago when his job
changed and became very pressurized.

Chris's Parkinson's has progressed in the past few years and his
abilities can vary from day to day. His main problems are with
freezing, muscular cramps, 'on–off' syndrome and speech that
varies in quality and deteriorates when he is 'off'. As a result he
says he tries to get as much as possible out when he is 'on' and
sometimes this causes his speech to become too fast for it to be
understood clearly. He is teaching himself to slow down when talking to counter this.

Chris has a complicated medication regimen involving several
different drugs, which have been adjusted several times as his
Parkinson's has progressed. He usually carries the entire day's allo-
cation in a small empty film container. When at home, a kitchen
timer is flexible enough to help him take his medication at the correct time. When he is out, he programmes his mobile phone alarm
and sets it on vibrate rather than a ringing tone when he is in meetings. He also keeps an updated list of his dosages and times on his
palm pilot as an *aide-mémoire*.

Diet is important in managing his medication and Chris is careful about what and when he eats in relation to his tablets. He eats
light foods and carbohydrates during the day and has his main protein in the evenings. He still drinks alcohol though he finds his
function is better if he limits this. He doesn't exercise as much as
he used to but on a good day can still swim several lengths of the
local gym pool and enjoys cycling along the river near his home.

Psychological aspects are also important to him. He knows that he went through a denial phase when he was first diagnosed. At some point however, he says, 'you have to confront yourself and determine what it means to have Parkinson's on a holistic level. You also have to tell people that you have Parkinson's. Once you have got through the denial phase, dealing with the rest of it is simpler.'

Five years ago Chris set up his own website (<http://www.young-parkinsons.org.uk>) as an important way of chronicling his experiences of Parkinson's and its progression. The aim of the website is to 'provide support through a connected world'. The contents include an account of his early symptoms and getting a diagnosis; information about his coping strategy, focusing on the symptoms that he finds crop up most often; and information and resources on Parkinson's. He also has a discussion forum. Chris enjoys doing the site and is pleased that so many people contact him, from all over the world, to say how much it has helped them, often at a difficult time when they have felt frightened and alone.

Chris has always been open about his Parkinson's, and has also given talks on Parkinson's at meetings for younger people, organized by the Parkinson's Disease Society; his doctor also sometimes asks him to participate in training for medical students.

Chris tries to be as positive as possible although there are times when this is not possible. When he has a bad day, he says, 'I just get on with things as best I can. I have lots of things to achieve while living on this earth and if I have to do this while living with Parkinson's, I will.'

The Cure Parkinson's Trust

Another example of finding your own self-help method is the Cure Parkinson's Trust, set up by four men who have Parkinson's. The Trust's aims include the drive towards a cure, and changing stereotypical misconceptions of Parkinson's while promoting a more positive outlook on the condition (see Useful addresses).

12

Young-onset Parkinson's disease

Parkinson's is often identified as a condition affecting only older people, despite the fact that one in seven of people diagnosed with it is under the age of 50 and one in 20 is under 40.

In the late 1980s, when I first worked at the Parkinson's Disease Society, the recognition of young-onset Parkinson's disease was very limited. Many younger people with Parkinson's I met at the time said that they had spent a long time going from one out-patients clinic to the next in search of a diagnosis. Many felt very isolated because the information resources on Parkinson's tended to focus on older people and it was also hard to meet other people with Parkinson's who were of a similar age.

Nowadays there is far more recognition and understanding of young-onset Parkinson's. In most cases, getting a diagnosis when younger seems to be quicker and there are now more resources, including those that have resulted from the development of the internet and e-mail. For many, the sense of being 'the only young one' with Parkinson's has been greatly reduced.

Medically, 'young-onset Parkinson's disease' describes the condition in someone who develops the symptoms of Parkinson's after the age of 21 and before the age of 40. In other contexts the term may be used to mean people of working age (that is, under 65). The term 'early-onset Parkinson's disease' is also sometimes used.

Most doctors believe that young-onset Parkinson's disease is idiopathic Parkinson's disease occurring at an earlier age, although some think it might be a different, related condition.

As with Parkinson's in older people, each younger person's experience of the condition will be different in terms of the nature and severity of symptoms, the rate of progression and the response to treatment.

In general, while symptoms are broadly the same at any age, there are some differences. Tremor tends to occur slightly less often in younger people but dystonic spasms (sustained abnormal postures, such as turning in or arching of the foot and toes) are more common. These often begin before the more typical Parkinson's features.

Younger people also seem to be more prone to depression. The

99

biological changes in the brain that Parkinson's causes play their part in this, but the main cause is the impact, psychologically and emotionally, that Parkinson's can have someone who is diagnosed when young.

Anecdotally, many younger women with Parkinson's report that their symptoms worsen before and during menstruation. Although there has been some preliminary research that supports this, more research on female hormones and their relationship to Parkinson's is needed.

The most significant differences between Parkinson's in younger people and older people lie in its medical management and in the factors that have an impact on a person's life as a result of being diagnosed at a younger age.

Juvenile parkinsonism

Very rarely, parkinsonism can occur in children and teenagers. The term 'juvenile Parkinson's disease' is used to describe parkinsonism that occurs before the age of 21. Although some people diagnosed with this condition turn out to have idiopathic Parkinson's disease, in many cases the symptoms turn out to be caused by rare inherited conditions, such as Segawa's syndrome (dopa-responsive dystonia), Huntington's disease with unusual features, or Wilson's disease.

Diagnosis of young-onset Parkinson's disease

There is no difference in the way that diagnosis is made in younger and older people. However, the differential diagnosis (the other possible medical conditions apart from Parkinson's that cause the symptoms being experienced) is particularly important when young-onset Parkinson's disease is suspected.

The doctor will be interested in any family history of either parkinsonism or essential tremor, because genetic links can be a factor. Wilson's disease also needs to be ruled out; this is a rare neurological condition that runs in families and has some parkinsonism symptoms such as tremor, rigidity and speech difficulties. It is caused by an increased accumulation of copper in the liver, brain and other parts of the body. Wilson's disease is a very treatable condition if caught early, and it can be identified from blood tests.

If you are reading this book because you think you might have young-onset Parkinson's disease, you need to discuss this with your GP and ask to be referred to a neurologist with a special interest in Parkinson's. (See also Chapter 4.)

Medical management

Although there is no difference in the treatments for younger and older people with Parkinson's, there are two important considerations in younger people:

- they will have to live with Parkinson's for much longer than most older people; and
- many have a more sensitive response to the drugs, particularly in terms of the side-effects.

Any decision about drugs needs to take into account your level of ability, quality of life, personal circumstances and needs. Because management is complicated, it is recommended that a neurologist should manage the care of all younger people with Parkinson's.

If the symptoms are mild, your doctor may advise against drugs immediately, waiting to see if symptoms develop.

When treatment is started, most doctors prefer to start younger people on dopamine agonists, anticholinergics or selegiline rather than levodopa, as these drugs tend to cause fewer side-effects than levodopa. They can often provide good symptom control to people in the early stages of Parkinson's, although in general they are not as effective as levodopa. As a result some people, especially those still working, sometimes choose to start taking levodopa immediately if it gives them better control of their symptoms.

When treated with levodopa, younger people often develop the side-effects associated with this drug, such as motor fluctuations and dyskinesia, quite early in treatment. If severe, these side-effects can have a considerable impact on daily activities. If levodopa is considered to be the best treatment for a younger person, the lowest dose possible will be prescribed in order to minimize potential side-effects.

Surgery can be an option for some younger people who have very disabling side-effects or who find the drugs ineffective. They are often better surgical candidates than older people because they are less likely to have other conditions that would complicate the procedures.

Psychological, emotional and social impact

Although it is difficult to cope with a diagnosis of Parkinson's at any age, for a younger person the implications are immense and the thought of coping with a future with Parkinson's can seem very daunting. You may be still working and have considerable financial commitments, such as a mortgage. You may also still be establishing relationships and wondering what effect Parkinson's might have on your emotional and sex life. You may be raising children and be concerned about the possible effects on them.

It is important to stress that with the right support, many young people do manage to lead happy and successful lives despite their Parkinson's. Sometimes doors can even open to new opportunities that were never dreamed of before, and some single people who despaired of finding a partner once they had Parkinson's have gone on to meet someone and marry them.

Never give up hope, no matter how difficult your circumstances may seem at times.

Support groups for younger people with Parkinson's

Many younger people with Parkinson's and their families find contact and involvement with a young-onset Parkinson's group extremely valuable in helping them to cope with Parkinson's (see Useful addresses).

Young Parkinson's Support Network (YPSN, formerly known as YAPP&Rs) is a group of the Parkinson's Disease Society.

The Parkinson's Association of Ireland has a group for younger people called PALS (see Useful addresses).

The American Parkinson Disease Association has a Young Parkinson's Disease group and produces a useful booklet.

Personal experiences

Michael J. Fox

'How could such a boyish-looking man be afflicted with a disease associated with older people?'[40]

This was the typical reaction of many people in 1998 when

Michael J. Fox, the Canadian film and television actor, then aged 37, announced that he had been diagnosed with Parkinson's seven years previously. Despite the extra dimension that his celebrity provides, his experiences, detailed in his autobiography *Lucky Man*, provide a classic account of young-onset Parkinson's.

Like many people, the first symptom he noticed was slight – some trembling in the little finger on his left hand, which eventually spread to the other fingers on the hand, followed by weakness in the left hand, stiffness in his shoulder and aching in the left side of his chest.

The diagnosis came when he was in his prime, developing a successful career as an actor and enjoying life with his wife Tracy and young son Sam. His early reactions to the diagnosis were disbelief and denial. He talks frankly in *Lucky Man* about how Parkinson's affected his self-esteem and how early methods of coping, including alcohol, had a detrimental effect on his family relationships.

Michael J. Fox eventually came to terms with Parkinson's and, although Parkinson's does cause him problems, he has managed to develop a positive attitude, maintaining a successful acting career and valuing his family and people with Parkinson's. Michael J. Fox has also used his celebrity to promote Parkinson's research through his Michael J. Fox Foundation, dedicated to ensuring the development of a cure for Parkinson's (see Useful addresses).

Karen

Karen lives in Leicester with her husband Nic and has had Parkinson's for 12 years, since the age of 33. At the time, she was a senior teacher of 3–11-year-olds, and after being diagnosed with Parkinson's she went on to become a deputy head, a post she held for four years until she retired early on medical grounds.

Karen had been having vague symptoms for about 12 months before being diagnosed – tiredness, a slight dragging of the left leg and tremor in one hand that came and went. At first after her diagnosis she didn't tell many people that she had Parkinson's, just her very supportive partner Nic, a few close friends and her colleagues at school, who were all supportive.

Karen, who knew little about Parkinson's disease, does not feel that she was given any information when she was diagnosed, and she found her local branch of the Parkinson's Disease Society herself. She feels that the internet, which was not available then, has subsequently made a tremendous difference to younger people with Parkinson's in terms of finding resources and making contact with others in a similar position.

The hardest aspects for Karen were being diagnosed so young and the loss of career opportunities with the subsequent economic consequences. When diagnosed, her immediate thought was that her teaching career would suffer. She doesn't know how she would have coped financially if she had been on her own. The inflexibility of the system that prevents her from working without jeopardizing her pension is particularly difficult for her. 'I have no peer group to relate to about this. I identified myself by my job and felt this was how others perceived me. Since retiring I have had to develop a new sense of self.' The effects of Parkinson's on her independence is also a worry although she still drives, has a very active life, and is planning a trip to India.

Karen believes in living for today. 'Anyone with a serious health condition has to consider how they exist,' she says, 'and it has to be about choosing to get on with life. I have gone "off" in some strange places, including an open-air amphitheatre in Verona, Italy, just as a performance of *Aida* was ending and everyone was fighting for the exits. When this happens, I just have to take some more pills and wait to go "on" again. I always make sure that I have my mobile phone and tablets with me. Humour plays a big part in coping with the condition. If you can laugh at things it is much easier to manage.'

Karen continues to contribute a great deal to her local community. She uses her teaching skills as a tutor on an adult voluntary literacy programme and the Expert Patients Programme (see Chapter 11). She is also chairwoman of the Young Parkinson's Support Network (YPSN).

Writing is another great interest. Using her knowledge as a teacher she has written *Our Mum has Parkinson's Disease*, a story book for children. She also enjoys writing poetry and is working on a radio play about Parkinson's. Writing was also useful to her during a period of clinical depression, as were a few sessions with an acupuncturist–counsellor. Massage also helps her to relax, and she feels that more complementary therapies should be available via the NHS because they can be very expensive, which is especially difficult for people on a limited income.

When I asked her what she would say to anyone newly diagnosed with Parkinson's, she said, 'There is life after Parkinson's. There can be a tendency to get into a symptom–pain–disease cycle that you need to take control and charge of. It is important to continue to live your life on a day-to-day basis. Don't let Parkinson's take you over. You will bump into a number of brick walls but you will learn to break through them.'

Jeff

Jeff is 45 and has been diagnosed with Parkinson's for three years. He lives with his wife Mary and two teenage children and still works five days a week as an agricultural worker. Jeff's main problems are with his hands curling up and with activities involving fine movements of the fingers. 'My symptoms get worse if I feel stressed so I try to think of other things to keep me going. I think that remaining positive is a big part of coping with Parkinson's. This is the card I have been dealt and I have to deal with it.'

Jeff started taking medication immediately and feels without it he would be incapacitated. He sees his neurologist every six months and also benefits from the advice of his Parkinson's disease nurse specialist. He likes the fact that his doctor involves him in decisions about his treatment.

Jeff is a member of his local young Parkinson's group and enjoys the contact with other people. 'I was a bit apprehensive when Mary and I first went but it felt like I was meeting people I hadn't met before. I didn't have to explain or apologize for myself. I like the informality and the opportunity to talk about experiences and feelings with friends in the same position.'

For newly diagnosed people, Jeff feels a user-friendly information pack would be helpful, providing a simple hands-on guide to what the condition is and reassuring you that you are not alone. 'It is difficult when you are newly diagnosed to make the phone calls to get the information you need, so anything that health and social care professionals can do to make this easier would be helpful.'

His message to other people who, like him, are diagnosed with Parkinson's at a young age is 'to remember that you are not on your own, that there are people out there like you and others who can provide you with support. When I discovered that, I felt that a ton of weight was lifted off me. If you let Parkinson's get to you, it will get you down. You should never say, "I can't do that because I have Parkinson's" but always try.'

13

Parkinson's disease in later life

Parkinson's is much more common in older people, starting at an average age of 60 years, and affecting one in 50 people over 80. The number of older people in the UK is increasing and therefore the incidence (number of new cases) and prevalence (absolute numbers of patients) of Parkinson's is also likely to rise considerably in the next 20–50 years.[41] Parkinson's that begins after the age of 70 is often referred to as 'late-onset Parkinson's disease'.

Diagnosing and treating Parkinson's in older people is complicated by the fact that many of the motor features of the condition are similar to the symptoms of many other diseases, especially arthritis, or may be mistaken for age-related changes. For instance, stiffness of muscles occurs with polymyalgia rheumatica, slowness in walking may occur with arthritis or poor eyesight, tremor may occur with anxiety or an overactive thyroid, and stooped posture may occur with osteoporosis.

The role of ageing in the development of Parkinson's is not entirely clear, though there is no doubt that it affects and interacts with Parkinson's symptoms and may be a contributing factor to the loss of dopamine in the brains of people with Parkinson's. However, ageing by itself probably doesn't entirely explain late-onset Parkinson's since some studies suggest that people who are very elderly (over 90) are less likely to have Parkinson's.

In older people with Parkinson's, problems with mobility and balance are often a particular feature that puts them at greater risk of having falls.

Depression and cognitive impairment, which are common in older people in general, are also common in Parkinson's and may be partly caused by the condition and partly by other coexisting factors. Cognitive impairment due to Parkinson's relates in part to duration of disease and the type of Parkinson's. At the age of 80, one in four people will have coexistent Alzheimer's.

The general health of older people is inclined to be less robust than that of younger people, and many older people have other health problems, such as diabetes, cardiovascular disease, arthritis and stroke, which complicate diagnosis, treatment and management. These other conditions can either produce symptoms similar to Parkinson's or exacerbate existing ones, so that it can be very difficult to distinguish between factors caused by Parkinson's and those that are the effect of these other conditions. Distinguishing between idiopathic Parkinson's disease and other forms of parkinsonism may also be more difficult as a result. Making this distinction is important because the proportion of parkinsonism not due to idiopathic Parkinson's disease increases with age and the response to therapy is different, depending on the type of parkinsonism (see Chapter 1).[42]

Drug-induced parkinsonism can also be common in older people, particularly if they are treated with drugs such as prochlorperazine (*Stemetil*), which is used to treat dizziness and nausea, and metoclopromide (*Maxolon*), used to prevent sickness and to treat indigestion (see Chapter 1).

Treatment

Whether or not to start drug treatment will be decided by the severity of disability – in other words, the nuisance value of symptoms for the person in question. All patients should be seen by a physiotherapist soon after diagnosis for advice regarding posture and exercise – this may be the only treatment needed in the early stages of Parkinson's. Other decisions about treatment will be influenced, not by age itself, but by any coexisting illnesses and any cognitive impairment (memory problems).

Response to any drug treatment changes with age. In general, older people metabolize and excrete drugs more slowly than younger people. This means that any given dose of drug lasts longer and has a greater effect in older people (alcohol is a good example of this – we get drunk more quickly and hangovers last longer and are more severe as we age!). If response to drug treatment is less than expected this is likely to be due to one of three reasons:

- an inadequate dose (undermedication);
- the symptoms are due to parkinsonism rather than true idiopathic Parkinson's disease; or
- there are other conditions, such as arthritis, contributing to the stiffness and slowness.

Neuropsychiatric problems (hallucinations, delusions and memory problems) associated with medication are more of a problem in older people because of a combination of factors:

- increased sensitivity to side-effects of medication with ageing;
- coexistent dementia (whether Alzheimer's or any other type of dementia); and
- the high prevalence of parkinsonism other than true idiopathic Parkinson's disease in older people (these conditions respond less well to dopaminergic therapy and people with them are more prone to develop the side-effects of these drugs).

All Parkinson's drugs have the potential for neuropsychiatric side-effects. The likelihood can be ranked by drug class: dopamine agonists more than anticholinergics more than MAOB inhibitors more than levodopa. Dopamine agonists and anticholinergics should be avoided in anyone with evidence of cognitive impairment. Anticholinergics are the best drugs for reducing tremor but need to be used cautiously, if at all, in older age because of their propensity to cause memory loss and confusion.

Treatment can also be complicated if the person is being treated for conditions other than Parkinson's, because the doctor has to guard against any contraindications or interactions that may occur if these medications are used together. (See Chapter 6.)

Older people are unlikely to be suitable candidates for neurosurgery. This is because their general health, coexisting conditions or cognitive impairment mean that the risks involved outweigh any potential benefits.

The complicated nature of late-onset Parkinson's means that a multidisciplinary team approach is important.

Older people are also more likely to be hospitalized, usually for reasons other than their Parkinson's, and it is important that the health-care staff know that the person has Parkinson's, as well as details of the drug regimen.

Carers of older people often have health problems themselves, making their role more difficult. Many older people live alone and so may need extra support to remain in their home. If they have many health needs and are struggling to cope, alternative accommodation may need to be considered. Some people experience financial hardship if they are trying to meet the extra costs of Parkinson's out of a pension, and transport can be a key issue for people living in a rural area.

Help is available from many sources. Have a look at Chapter 5 for more information on health and social care professionals, at Chapter 8 for information on financial help and transport, and at Chapter 11 for information about living alone and safety.

Many of the local branches of the Parkinson's Disease Society have community support workers who can provide advice, as can voluntary organizations such as Age Concern, Help the Aged, and Counsel and Care (see Useful addresses).

Personal experiences

Ken

Ken is 73 and has had Parkinson's for 13 years. He worked as a painter and decorator for 46 years but retired from work in 1992 when he was diagnosed with cervical spondylosis. Ken lives with his wife of 53 years, Peggy, and they have a son and daughter.

Ken's main problems are to do with his mobility, especially walking. He finds any complicated actions, such as turning, very difficult. Putting on socks, tying laces, managing zips and shaving are also hard for him, because of problems with fine movements of the fingers. He has a lot of tremor, which gets worse if he is nervous or upset and this can be embarrassing when it happens in public. 'Parkinson's is very unpredictable and tiring. I feel sometimes like two people. One minute I can be my "normal self" but the next minute I am a different person, unable to do what I was freely doing before. It is like being switched on and off. Planning things in advance is impossible and we have to take every day as it comes.'

Ken has tried various drugs to treat his Parkinson's. With some he experienced hallucinations and panic attacks. He takes his tablets three times a day and says that it is very important that he should take them at the particular times that suit his needs. He says his best time of the day is the first hour in the morning and he always takes Peggy a cup of tea when he gets up. One of Ken's great loves is canaries – he has shown them and judged at competitions most of his life. Although at one time he had about 80 birds, nowadays he has about 10 and keeps up his interest with the help of a friend who takes him to the canary shows.

Ken's Parkinson's is complicated by the fact that three years ago he had a stroke, which has affected the same side as his Parkinson's. At the time of the stroke, he couldn't move his right hand or any of his right side. For a while his tremors seemed to be less obvious after the stroke but they are now starting to come back. He finds it hard to know whether some of the symptoms he has are caused by the Parkinson's or the stroke. 'My general health is about average compared with other people of the same age who have Parkinson's and have had it for the same length of time. I have lost a lot of confidence, which makes it harder to meet a lot of new people. However, the support I had from the nursing staff and physiotherapists when I was in hospital was brilliant. I have also benefited from the advice of two Parkinson's disease nurse specialists, who have been very helpful and understanding with any problems I have encountered between appointments with the neurologist.'

Ken and Peggy say they cope with Parkinson's together. Keeping a sense of humour is important. Transport can be a problem now that they have both given up driving and they rely a lot on taxis, which can be expensive. Shops can be difficult to manage, especially if there is no seat for Ken to sit down on if he needs to. Supermarkets with facilities for people with disabilities are the easiest for Ken to manoeuvre around.

Peggy says she hasn't been provided with much support to help her cope as a carer but has learnt 'on the job'. She says, 'I think it is important to encourage people with Parkinson's to do as much as they can for themselves and not to do too much for them, especially early on. Ken is strong-willed and won't give into things. He likes to do things himself if he can. It is important to take each day as it comes and not to think every day is going to be a bad day.'

Avril

Avril is 72 and was diagnosed with Parkinson's about six years ago. She and her husband, David, have three children and two grandchildren.

Her diagnosis of Parkinson's was made during an appointment for another medical condition and she was referred to a neurologist, whom she saw within two or three weeks. She says she suspected that something was wrong because she had been feeling dreadful for some time with a lot of shoulder and back trouble. Some months before her diagnosis she was shaking so much during a routine medical test that the nurse suggested Avril mention this to the doctor – he said it was age. David thought she might have Parkinson's because he had a friend with it and spotted some similarity in Avril's walking.

Avril felt upset and frightened when told she had Parkinson's, particularly as she went into the consultation on her own, and wasn't given any real explanation of what Parkinson's was, only that there was help available but no cure. Her symptoms also fluctuated at first, so that at times she was sure that a mistake had been made in the diagnosis. 'What frustrates me most about Parkinson's is the lack of independence and mobility. I don't like not being in control. I can't walk far and can't go into town without someone with me.'

As soon as she was diagnosed, Avril started on medication and is now on five tablets a day. Although the awful sense she had before her diagnosis of 'wading through another world' has gone, she doesn't think her drugs help with the balance or walking difficulties that she has.

In addition to Parkinson's, Avril has other health problems, including heart problems and type 2 diabetes, which is controlled by diet. 'The symptoms of each are mixed in together and I find it hard to separate out what is caused by which condition,' she says. Avril had a heart bypass a few years ago, after unsuccessful angioplasty. She says, 'The stress of the operation has made my Parkinson's worse and I took a long time to recover. It's difficult to know what is the result of the heart problems and the operation and what is Parkinson's, but anyone who is having an operation who has Parkinson's should be prepared for recovery to take longer.'

Although she was well treated in hospital, she feels the aftercare could have been improved. 'You are just left to get on with it. No one tells you what to do or what help you are going to need. David had problems parking at the hospital when he came to pick me up and we had to hire a wheelchair ourselves from the British Red Cross.'

Avril and David cope with Parkinson's together and feel that they 'stagger on from day to day. We enjoy meeting our friends at the local Parkinson's branch for a moan and a laugh. It's important to be positive and not sit there thinking you are going into a decline. Make the best of what you can and find your own way of coping.'

14

Carers, families and friends

If you are the partner, relative or close friend of someone with Parkinson's, you are probably wondering what changes their diagnosis is going to bring to your life as well as theirs. There is no doubt that Parkinson's will probably mean making some adjustments to your life, and no matter how much you love the person with Parkinson's and want to support him or her, it is natural to have questions about the sort of care you are going to have to provide and how you are going to cope with this.

Given the idiosyncratic nature of Parkinson's, it is very difficult to say exactly what sort of support you might have to provide. So much depends on the symptoms; how these affect day-to-day life; what other medical conditions the person has; the person's attitude to the condition; how independent he or she wants to be; the relationship you have with each other; and whether you live together or are providing care from a distance.

In the early stages, most people with Parkinson's do not require too much physical help, unless they have other conditions that complicate the situation. They may, however, need a lot of emotional support, especially at diagnosis, often a particularly difficult time. This can also be hard for family members and friends, who may have similar feelings to the person with Parkinson's – difficulty coming to terms with Parkinson's and fears about the future. Sometimes the carer and person with Parkinson's can find themselves at different stages in accepting the diagnosis. One person (and it might be either the person with the condition or the carer) may still be denying Parkinson's while the other is eagerly trying to learn everything possible about the condition. The one who has accepted that Parkinson's is now part of his or her life may want to talk about Parkinson's to the other, who is still in denial and is therefore resistant to any suggestions or dialogue.

As their Parkinson's develops, many people start to require help with practical tasks, and relatives and friends can find that more of their time is taken up with providing support. This support is often described as 'caring' and the person providing the care as 'a carer'. Although providing this support is often something that people want to do, it can be very demanding and impinge in many ways on the carer's life. If you are a carer it is important that you take advantage of the many carers' resources and services that are available.

Although the needs of each carer and the person being cared for will be different, there are several key things that are essential to the well-being of most carers. These include:

- ensuring the well-being of the person they are caring for;
- information and education – about the health condition in question (in this case Parkinson's), about being a carer, about practical aspects of care (such as moving and handling the person) and about the help available;
- services to help them with caring that also allow them to have a life of their own and ensure that their own health and well-being is maintained – such as respite care services and financial benefits;
- a say in the provision of these services; and
- opportunities to meet others in a similar position.

Resources to help carers

Carer's assessment

Your local social services department can arrange support services for people who need help to live independently in the community and will first carry out a 'needs' or 'care' assessment. Under the Carers and Children Act 2000 a carer is also entitled to have an assessment of his or her own needs.

Services are largely dependent on the area where you live but might include support in your home to help you with caring tasks or housework; day care or respite care services to give you a break; equipment or alterations to your house; or opportunities for social contacts and leisure, for example carers' groups.

Although the assessment will be free, who pays for any services subsequently recommended depends on your financial situation and the eligibility criteria for service provision in your area. Don't assume that any health professionals that are involved in the care of the person with Parkinson's will automatically suggest a carer's assessment if you need one. If you think you could benefit from one, ask for one via your local social services. The phone number will be listed in your local telephone directory under the local authority, or your GP's surgery should be able to provide you with the details.

Carer's allowance

The carer's allowance is a taxable financial benefit that is available to informal carers, aged 16 or over, who regularly spend more than 35 hours a week caring for someone who is severely disabled.

Carers' organizations

There are several carers' organizations that campaign for carers' rights and services. These include Carers UK and the Princess Royal Trust for Carers (which has local carers' centres across the UK where carers can obtain information and advice <http://www.carers.org>). (See Useful addresses.)

Some Primary Care Trusts also have carers' workers. Your GP or local Patient Advice and Liaison Service should be able to advise you what is available in your local area.

Carers' emergency cards and schemes

Carers' emergency cards can be obtained from Carers UK and are similar to an organ donation card. They identify you as a carer and allow you to give details of people who can be contacted in the event of an emergency or accident, to ensure that the person you are caring for is looked after.

Some local authorities and carers' centres also run carer emergency schemes. Carers carry a card that shows the telephone number of the scheme and a unique PIN. If there is an emergency, the carer or someone else can call the scheme and using the unique PIN the operator can look up and activate the emergency plan to ensure replacement care.

Employment

The Carers (Equal Opportunities Act) 2004 aims to tackle barriers that carers face in accessing employment, education and leisure. Carers UK is the lead partner in a scheme called Action for Carers and Employment, which aims to raise awareness of the barriers facing carers who want to work and to test and promote ways of supporting them.

Advice on employment is also available from your local Princess Royal Trust for Carers centre. Some centres have also initiated courses looking specifically at carers and employment issues.

Respite care

Caring can be exhausting, and regular breaks can help you cope, whether it's a few hours a week, a longer holiday break or regular care from a day centre or other facility. This is often called respite care and can take many forms.

Carers UK and your local Princess Royal Trust for Carers centre can provide you with more information about respite care. Your local social services should also be able to tell you about what is available in your area.

Courses for carers

Some of the carers I talked to while writing this book said that it would have helped them to have been able to go on a course for carers to help them understand more about what might be involved and where to get help.

City and Guilds, one of the UK's leading providers of vocational qualifications, has developed an on-line learning resource for carers, called Learning for Living (<http://www.learning-for-living.co.uk>).

Many Princess Royal Trust for Carers centres also run courses, and some therapists in your local hospital may run courses on aspects of caring such as lifting and handling.

Resources for carers of people with Parkinson's

The Parkinson's Disease Society has several resources for carers of people with Parkinson's, including a carers' guide and an annual *Holidays and Respite Care Guide*. They also provide advice and support to carers and campaign for recognition and services for carers.

15

The future

In the past 20–30 years, there have been enormous advances in the management of Parkinson's. There will be many more in the next few years that will, it is to be hoped, result in new and better therapies, improved quality of life, ways of preventing Parkinson's progressing and – ultimately – a cure.

Let me demonstrate how rapidly developments can move in the space of 20 years. When I started working at the Parkinson's Disease Society in the late 1980s, the drug treatments available were limited. Although levodopa had been in use since the end of the 1960s, doctors were still learning about its long-term effects. During my employment at the Parkinson's Disease Society (1987–2004), at least six new drugs were developed as treatments for Parkinson's – pramipexole (*Mirapexin*), ropinirole (*Requip*), cabergoline (*Cabaser*), entacapone (*Comtess*), tolcapone (*Tasmar*) and the combined co-careldopa–entacapone drug, *Stalevo*. Interest in apomorphine (*Apo-go*) was also revived about this time when doctors discovered that the sickness that this drug caused, which had prevented its use, could be overcome by prescribing an antiemetic (anti-sickness) drug, domperidone, with it. All these treatments have made an immense difference to the lives of thousands of people with Parkinson's and have increased considerably the range of treatment options that doctors can use. A further drug, rasagiline (*Azilect*) was licensed in 2005.

Many other possible drug treatments are currently being researched. Areas of interest include:

- alternative delivery systems such as nasal sprays, gels and patches – it is possible that a skin patch containing a dopamine agonist called rotigotine may be licensed in 2006;
- treatments based on other systems and substances in the brain, apart from dopamine, that may be involved in Parkinson's;
- drugs that may enhance the effects of levodopa or reduce the side-effects that can occur with its long-term use; and
- antioxidants.

In the past few years there has also been a resurgence of interest in surgery. Some techniques, discussed in Chapter 7, show promise as treatments for some people who have advanced Parkinson's. Stem cell research, although now in its infancy, may also in time lead to exciting new developments in Parkinson's treatment.

Gene therapy is another promising area of Parkinson's research. This technique involves using genes as drugs, either to introduce normal genes into the body in order to overcome certain defects or to deliver substances that can affect biochemical functions that cause diseases.

Understanding of Parkinson's, biologically and chemically, has also grown tremendously. To do this, researchers need to compare the functions of a normal brain with that of a Parkinson's brain. Tissue banks, such as the UK Parkinson's Disease Society Tissue Bank in London (see Useful addresses), collect and store tissue that has been donated by people with Parkinson's and controls (i.e. those without Parkinson's). These donations can then be used in the UK and internationally to further Parkinson's research into the processes of the brain that are involved and into new treatments.

There has also been greater recognition of the social, psychological and emotional impact of Parkinson's, and more research is now focused on quality-of-life issues, rehabilitation and care. One of the most significant developments in this area has been Parkinson's disease nurse specialists. Other projects have looked at the importance of multidisciplinary management involving several different types of health and social care professionals, psychological aspects of Parkinson's, carers' issues, and the role that occupational therapy, physiotherapy and occupational therapy can play in the management of Parkinson's.

The internet and e-mail, which were not available in the late 1980s, has made exchanging information and experiences far easier, not just for people living with the condition but also doctors and researchers involved in Parkinson's work. We can only guess at the kinds of technological advances that may be made in the next 20 years to improve communication even further.

Whatever your reason for reading this book, I hope that its contents and the stories of the people with Parkinson's and their families that appear in it have reassured you that there is life after a diagnosis of Parkinson's and that there is always hope for the future.

Further reading

Rasheda Ali (2005) *I'll Hold Your Hand so You Won't Fall Down*, Weybridge, Surrey, Merit Publishing International. (For children.)

Svend Andersen (2002) *Health is Between Your Ears: Living with a chronic illness*, Hornslet, Denmark, Hornslet Bogtrykkeri.

Glenna Wotton Atwood (1991) *Living Well with Parkinson's*, Chichester, West Sussex, John Wiley and Sons.

Barbara Blake-Krebs and Linda Herman (2002) *When Parkinson's Strikes Early: Voices, choices, resources and treatment*, Alameda, California, Hunter House Publishers.

Painton Cowen (2003) *Six Days: The story of the making of the Chester Cathedral Creation Window*, Bristol, Alistair Sawday Publishing. (Window created by Rosalind Grimshaw.)

Sidney Dorros (1998) *Parkinson's: A patient's view*, London, Class Publishing. (British edition with an introduction by Les Essex.)

Michael J. Fox (2002) *Lucky Man*, London, Ebury Press.

Karen Gavin (2000) *Our Mum has Parkinson's Disease*, London, Parkinson's Disease Society. (For children.)

Dennis Greene, Joan Blessington Snyder and Craig L. Kendall, *Voices from the Parking Lot: Parkinson's insights and perspectives*, Princeton, New Jersey, The Parkinson's Alliance.

R. K. Griffiths and E. H. Coene (eds) (2000) *Parkinson's Disease Self-Care Manual/CD-ROM*, September Foundation. (See <http://www.pdupdate.org> for more information.)

David A. Grimes (2004) *Parkinson's Disease: A guide to treatments, therapies and controlling symptoms*, London, Constable and Robinson.

Marjan Jahanshahi and C. David Marsden (2000) *Parkinson's Disease: A self-help guide*, New York, Demos Medical Publishing.

Abraham Lieberman with Marcia McCall (2003) *100 Questions and Answers about Parkinson's Disease*, Sudbury, Massachusetts, Jones and Bartlett Publishers.

Bridget McCall, Adrian Williams and Marie Oxtoby (2004) *Parkinson's at Your Fingertips*, 3rd edition, London, Class Publishing.

Oliver Sacks (1991) *Awakenings*, Basingstoke, Hampshire, Picador.

Harvey Sagar (2002) *The Parkinson's Disease Handbook*, London, Vermillion Press.

Jacob Sage and Roger C. Duvoisin (2001) *Parkinson's Disease: A guide for patient and family*, Philadelphia, Lippincott Williams and Wilkins.

For health professionals

Carl E. Clarke (2001) *Parkinson's Disease in Practice*, London, RSM Press.
Christopher G. Clough, K. Ray Chaudhuri and Kapil D. Sethi (2003) *Parkinson's Disease* (Fast Facts series), Oxford, Health Press.
Jolyon Meara and William C. Koller (eds) (2000) *Parkinson's Disease and Parkinsonism in the Elderly*, Cambridge, Cambridge University Press.
Lesley Swinn (2005) *Parkinson's Disease: Theory and practice for nurses*, Chichester, Whurr Publishers.

Useful addresses

Organizations
Parkinson's specific

American Parkinson Disease Association
135 Parkinson Avenue
Staten Island
New York
NY 10305
Tel.: 1 800 223 2732
Website: www.apdaparkinson.org
Email: apda@apdaparkinson.org
Handbook on young-onset Parkinson's: www.apdaparkinson.org/data/
booklets

European Parkinson's Disease Association
Registered office:
Avenue Nestor Plissart 4
1040 Brussels
Belgium

Secretary-General:
4 Golding Road
Sevenoaks
Kent
TN13 3NJ
Tel.: 01732 457683
Website: www.epda.eu.com

Michael J. Fox Foundation for Parkinson's Research
Grand Central Station
PO Box 4777
New York
NY 10163
Tel.: 1 800 708 7644
Website: www.michaeljfox.org

Parkinson's Association of Ireland
Carmichael House
North Brunswick Street
Dublin 7
Eire
Tel.: Freephone 1 800 359 359 (9.30 am to 3 pm, Monday to Friday)
Website: www.parkinsons.ie

Email: parkinsonsireland@eircom.net
PALS (website for younger people):
http://gofree.indigo.ie/~pdpals/pdn1.htm

Parkinson's Disease Society
215 Vauxhall Bridge Road
London SW1V 1EJ
Tel.: 020 7931 8080
Advisory Freephone Line: 0808 800 0303 (9.30 am to 5.30 pm, Monday to
Friday)
Website: www.parkinsons.org.uk
For young people www.young-parkinsons.org.uk or www.youngonset-
parkinsons.org.uk
Email: enquiries@parkinsons.org.uk

Special Parkinson's Research Interest Group (SPRING)
PO Box 440
Horsham
West Sussex RH13 0YE
Tel.: 01483 281307
Website: http://spring.parkinsons.org.uk
Email: info@spring.parkinsons.org.uk

UK Parkinson's Disease Society Tissue Bank
Division of Neuroscience & Mental Health
Imperial College London
Faculty of Medicine
Charing Cross Campus
Fulham Palace Road
London W6 8RF
Tel.: 020 8383 4917
Website: www.parkinsonstissuebank.org.uk
Email: pdbank@imperial.ac.uk

Disease specific

Alzheimer's Society
Gordon House
Greencoat Place
London SW1P 1PH
Tel.: 020 7306 0606
Website: www.alzheimers.org.uk
Email: enquiries@alzheimers.org.uk

Alzheimer Scotland – Action on Dementia
22 Drumsheugh Gardens
Edinburgh EH3 7RN
Tel.: 0131 243 1453
Website: www.alzscot.org
Email: alzheimer@alzscot.org

British Brain and Spine Foundation
7 Winchester House
Cranmer Road
Kennington Park
London SW9 6EJ
Tel.: 020 7793 5900
Helpline: 0808 808 1000 (9 am to 1 pm, Monday, Tuesday, Thursday, Friday; 10 am to 6 pm Wednesday)
Website: www.bbsf.org.uk
Email: helpline@brainandspine.org.uk

The National Tremor Foundation
Harold Wood Hospital (DSC)
Gubbins Lane
Romford
Essex RM3 0AR
Tel.: 0800 328 8046 (freephone)
Website: www.tremor.org.uk
Email: tremorfoundation@aol.com

The Pick's Disease Support Group
8 Brooksby Close
Oadby
Leicester LE2 5AB
Helpline: 0845 458 3208
Website: www.pdsg.org.uk
Email: info@pdsg.org.uk

The Progressive Supranuclear Palsy (PSP Europe) Association
The Old Rectory
Wappenham
Towcester
Northants NN12 8SQ
Tel.: 01327 860299
Website: www.pspeur.org
Email: psp@pspeur.org

The Sarah Matheson Trust for Multiple System Atrophy
Pickering Unit
St Mary's Hospital
Praed Street
London W2 1NY
Tel.: 020 7886 1520 (9.30 am to 4.30 pm, Monday to Friday)
Website: www.msaweb.co.uk
Email (general enquiries): office@msaweb.co.uk

The Stroke Association
240 City Road
London EC1V 2PR
Helpline: 0845 303 3100
Website: www.stroke.org.uk
Email: info@stroke.org.uk

Wilson's Disease Association International
1802 Brookside Drive
Wooster
OH 44691
USA
Website: www.wilsonsdisease.org
Email: info@wilsonsdisease.org

Other organizations

AbilityNet Central England
PO Box 94
Warwick CV34 5WS
Freephone helpline: 0800 269 545
Website: www.abilitynet.org.uk

Charity that provides expertise on computing and accessing information
technology for people with disabilities.

Age Concern England
Astral House
1268 London Road
London SW16 4ER
Free information line: 0800 00 99 66 (8 am to 7 pm, seven days a week)
Website: www.ageconcern.org.uk

Birmingham Clinical Trials Unit (for information on PD Med and PD Surg)
Park Grange
1 Somerset Road
Edgbaston
Birmingham B15 2RR
Tel.: 0121 687 2315
Website: www.pdmed.bham.ac.uk

The British Association for Counselling and Psychotherapy
BACP House
35–37 Albert Street
Rugby
Warwickshire CV21 2SG
Tel.: 0870 443 5252
Website: www.bacp.co.uk
Email: bacp@bacp.co.uk

The British Association/College of Occupational Therapists
106–114 Borough High Street
Southwark
London SE1 1LB
Tel.: 020 7357 6480
Website: www.baot.org.uk

British Complementary Medicine Association
PO Box 5122
Bournemouth BH8 0WG
Tel.: 0845 345 5977
Website: www.bcma.co.uk

British Dietetic Association
5th Floor, Charles House
148/9 Great Charles Street
Queensway
Birmingham B3 3HT
Tel.: 0121 200 8080
Website: www.bda.uk.com
Email: info@bda.uk.com

The Calvert Trust
Barnstaple Centre: Tel.: 01598 763221
Keswick Centre: Tel.: 017687 72255
Kielder Centre: Tel.: 01434 250232
Website: www.calvert-trust.org.uk

Provides outdoor-activity holidays for people with disabilities, their families, friends and carers.

Carers UK
20–25 Glasshouse Yard
London EC1A 4JT
CarersLine: 0808 808 7777 (10 am to 12 noon and 2 pm to 4 pm, Wednesday and Thursday)
Tel.: 020 7490 8818
Website: www.carersuk.org
Email: info@carersuk.org

Centre for Accessible Environments
70 South Lambeth Road
London SW8 1RL
Tel.: 020 7840 0125
Website: www.cae.org.uk
Email: info@cae.org.uk

Charity Search
25 Portview Road
Avonmouth
Bristol BS11 9LD
Tel.: 0117 982 4060

Provides a free service to assist elderly people who are in financial difficulty to find a charity that might be able to help.

Chartered Society of Physiotherapists
14 Bedford Row
London WC1R 4ED
Tel.: 020 7833 2181
Website: www.csp.org.uk

Citizens Advice (NACAB: the National Association of Citizens Advice Bureaux)
Myddelton House
115–123 Pentonville Road
London N1 9LZ
Tel.: 020 7833 2181
Website: www.adviceguide.org.uk

City & Guilds/Learning for Living
1 Giltspur Street
London EC1A 9DD
Tel.: 020 7294 2800
Website: www.learning-for-living.co.uk
Email: enquiry@cityandguilds.com

An on-line learning programme designed specifically for unpaid carers.

Complementary Medical Association
Tel.: 0845 129 8434
Website: www.the-cma.org.uk

Counsel and Care
Twyman House
16 Bonny Street
London NW1 9PG
Tel.: 020 7241 8555
Website: www.counselandcare.org.uk
Email: advice@counselandcare.org.uk

Department for Work and Pensions
DWP Public Enquiry Office
Tel.: 020 7712 2171
Helpline: 0800 88 22 00
Website: www.dwp.gov.uk
Jobcentre Plus website: www.jobcentreplus.gov.uk

The Depression Alliance
212 Spitfire Studios
63–71 Collier Street
London N1 9BE
Tel.: 0845 123 23 20
Website: www.depressionalliance.org
Email: information@depressionalliance.org

The Directory of Social Change
24 Stephenson Way
London NW1 2DP
Tel.: 020 7391 4800
Helpline: 08450 77 77 07
Website: www.dsc.org.uk
Email: info@dsc.org.uk

The Disability Rights Commission
DRC Helpline
Freepost MID 02164
Stratford-upon-Avon
CV37 9BR
Helpline: 08457 622 633 (8 am to 8 pm, Monday to Friday)
Textphone (Minicom): 08457 622 644
Website: www.drc-gb.org

Disabled Living Centres Council
Assist UK
Redbank House
4 St Chad's Street
Cheetham
Manchester M8 8QA
Tel.: 0870 770 2866
Website: www.dlcc.org.uk
Email: general.info@assist-uk.org

Disabled Living Foundation
380–384 Harrow Road
London W9 2HU
Tel.: 020 7289 6111
Helpline: 0845 130 9177 (10 am to 4 pm, Monday to Friday)
Website: www.dlf.org.uk
Fact sheets: www.dlf.org.uk/factsheets

Disabled Persons Railcard Office
PO Box 163
Newcastle-upon-Tyne NE12 8WX
Tel.: 0191 218 8103
Text phone: 0191 269 0304

USEFUL ADDRESSES

EXCEL 2000
1A North Street
Sheringham
Norfolk NR26 8LW
Tel.: 01263 825670 (9 am to 5 pm, Monday to Friday)
Website: www.excel2000.org.uk

Aims to help improve the quality of life for those living with physical, mental or emotional impairment. The method includes movement and music and exercise. Audio CDs are available and workshops and training courses are offered to instructors.

Gardening for Disabled Trust
Hayes Farmhouse
Hayes Lane
Peasmarsh
Rye
East Sussex TN31 6XR
Website: www.gardeningfordisabledtrust.org.uk

Help the Aged
207–221 Pentonville Road
London N1 9UZ
Tel.: 020 7278 1114
Seniorline: 0808 800 6565
Website: www.helptheaged.org.uk
Email: info@helptheaged.org.uk

Holiday Care
Tourism for All
The Hawkins Suite
Enham Place
Enham Alamein
Andover SP11 6JS
Tel.: 0845 124 9971
Website: www.holidaycare.org.uk
Email: info@tourismforall.org.uk

Mind
15–19 Broadway
London E15 4BQ
Tel.: 020 8519 2122
Helpline (Mindinfoline): 08457 660163
Website:www.mind.org.uk
Email: contact@mind.org.uk

Motability
Goodman House
Station Approach
Harlow
Essex CM20 2ET
Tel.: 01279 635999 (8.45 am to 5.15 pm, Monday to Friday)

National Pharmacy Association
Mallison House
38–42 St Peter's Street
St Albans
Herts AL1 3NP
Tel.: 01727 832161
Patient website: www.askyourpharmacist.co.uk

NHS Direct (England and Northern Ireland)
Tel.: 0845 4647
Minicom: 0845 606 4647
Website: www.nhs.direct.nhs.uk

Occupational Therapists in Independent Practice
Tel.: 0800 389 4873
Website: www.otip.co.uk

The Patients Association
PO Box 935
Harrow
Middlesex HA1 3YJ
Helpline: 0845 608 4455 (10 am to 4 pm, Monday to Friday)
Website: www.patients-association.org.uk
Email: mailbox@patients-association.com

The Pension Service
Tel.: 0845 60 60 265 (8 am to 8 pm, Monday to Friday)
Website: www.thepensionservice.gov.uk

RADAR (The Royal Association for Disability and Rehabilitation)
12 City Forum
250 City Road
London EC1V 8AF
Tel.: 020 7250 3222
Website: www.radar.org.uk
Email: radar@radar.org.uk

The Royal College of Psychiatrists
17 Belgrave Square
London SW1X 8PG
Tel.: 020 7235 2351
Website: www.rcpsych.ac.uk

The Royal College of Speech and Language Therapists
2 White Hart Yard
London SE1 1NX
Tel.: 020 7378 1200
Website: www.rcslt.org.uk

The Royal Pharmaceutical Society of Great Britain
1 Lambeth High Street
London SE1 7JN
Tel.: 020 7234 8620
Website: www.rpsgb.org.uk
Email: enquiries@rpsgb.org

The Society of Chiropodists and Podiatrists
1 Fellmonger's Path
Tower Bridge Road
London SE1 3LY
Tel.: 020 7234 8620
Website: www.feetforlife.org

Thrive
Sir Geoffrey Udall Centre
Beech Hill
Reading RG7 2AT
Tel.: 0118 988 5688
Website: www.thrive.org.uk

Aims for a positive change in the lives of disabled and disadvantaged people through gardening.

Tourism for All
C/o Vitalise
Shap Road Industrial Estate
Shap Road
Kendal
Cumbria LA9 6NZ
Tel.: 0845 124 9971
Website: www.tourismforall.org.uk
Email: info@tourismforall.org.uk

Tripscope
Tel. and Minicom: 08457 58 56 41
Website: www.tripscope.org.uk

Helpline service advising on transport issues for people with disabilities.

UK Online
Tel.: 0800 77 1234
Website: www.direct.gov.uk

Online directory of a variety of public services.

Websites

Art for Parkinson's
www.artforparkinsons.org.uk

Awakenings – Parkinson's Disease
www.parkinsonsdisease.com

Bandolier
www.jr2.ox.ac.ik/bandolier
Monthly newsletter about evidence-based healthcare.

Chris Chapman
www.young-parkinsons.org.uk

Website for young people living and coping with Parkinson's.

The Cure Parkinson's Trust
www.cureparkinsons.org.uk

Embarrassing Problems
www.embarrassingproblems.com

The Expert Patients Programme
Helpline: 0845 606 6040
Website: www.expertpatients.nhs.uk

The Guardian
www.guardian.co.uk

Articles by David Beresford, 'Bad Science', and Professor Edzard Ernst's columns.

learndirect
Tel.: 0800 100 900
Website: www.learndirect.co.uk

National Parkinson Foundation (Florida, USA)
www.parkinson.org

Parkinson's Disease Foundation (New York, USA)
www.pdf.org

P-I-E-N-O
www.parkinsons-information-exchange-network-online.com

International site for people with Parkinson's.

Quackwatch
www.quackwatch.org

Notes

1 A. Lieberman (2003) *100 Questions and Answers about Parkinson's Disease*, Sudbury, Massachusetts, Jones and Bartlett Publishers, p. 39.

2 B. Ridha, *Corticobasal Degeneration*, available on the Pick's Disease Support Group website (<http://www.pdsg.org.uk>) (accessed June 2005).

3 Based on I. McKeith, *What is Dementia with Lewy Bodies?*, available on the Alzheimer's Society website (<http://www.alzheimers.org.uk>) (accessed June 2005).

4 B. McCall (2004) *Drug-induced Parkinson's Disease* (Parkinson's Disease Society Information Sheet FS38) London, Parkinson's Disease Society.

5 M. Jahanshahi, C. D. Marsden (2000) *Parkinson's Disease: A self-help guide*, New York, Demos Medical Publishing, p. 22.

6 Based on information on the National Tremor Foundation website (<http://www.tremor.org.uk>) (accessed September 2005).

7 Based on information on the Sarah Matheson Trust for Multiple System Atrophy website (<http://www.msaweb.co.uk>) (accessed September 2005).

8 M. Jahanshahi, C. D. Marsden (2000) *Parkinson's Disease: A self-help guide*, New York, Demos Medical Publishing, p. 20.

9 A. Lieberman (2003) *100 Questions and Answers about Parkinson's Disease*, Sudbury, Massachusetts, Jones and Bartlett Publishers, p. 39.

10 B. McCall (Autumn 2004) 'Do strokes cause Parkinsonism?', *The Parkinson*, Parkinson's Disease Society, p. 23.

11 C. E. Clarke (2001) *Parkinson's Disease in Practice*, London, RSM Press, p. 1.

12 M. Jahanshahi, C. D. Marsden (2000) *Parkinson's Disease: A self-help guide*, New York, Demos Medical Publishing, p. 3.

13 *One in Twenty: An information pack for younger people with Parkinson's* (2002) (Booklet B77), London, Parkinson's Disease Society, Introduction.

14 C. G. Clough, K. R. Chaudhuri, K. D. Sethi (2003) *Parkinson's Disease*, Oxford, Health Press (Fast Facts series), p. 9.

15 C. E. Clarke (2001) *Parkinson's Disease in Practice*, London, RSM Press p. 1.

16 L. Swinn (2005) 'Pathogenesis of Parkinson's disease', in L. Swinn (ed) *Parkinson's Disease: Theory and practice for nurses*, Chichester, Whurr Publishers, p. 4.

17 C. E. Clarke (2001) *Parkinson's Disease in Practice*, London, RSM Press, p. 8.

18 M. Jahanshahi, C. D. Marsden (2000) *Parkinson's Disease: A self-help guide*, New York, Demos Medical Publishing, p. 22.

19 C. E. Clarke (2001) *Parkinson's Disease in Practice*, London, RSM Press, pp. 5–6.
20 C. Cosgrove (2003) *Antioxidants* (Parkinson's Disease Society Information Sheet FS67), London, Parkinson's Disease Society.
21 C. Cosgrove (2002) *Co-enzyme Q10* (Parkinson's Disease Society Information Sheet FS74), London, Parkinson's Disease Society.
22 L. Melton (2004) *A glimpse into the latest research on Parkinson's disease* (Parkinson's Disease Society Science in Progress article), London, Parkinson's Disease Society.
23 L. Swinn (2005) 'Pathogenesis of Parkinson's disease', in *Parkinson's Disease: Theory and practice for nurses*, Chichester, Whurr Publishers, p. 10.
24 Based on C. Cosgrove (2004) *Freezing* (Parkinson's Disease Society Information Sheet FS63), London, Parkinson's Disease Society.
25 C. Cosgrove (2004) *Muscle Cramps and Dystonia* (Parkinson's Disease Society Information Sheet FS43), London, Parkinson's Disease Society.
26 Based on C. Cosgrove (2003) *Fatigue* (Parkinson's Disease Society Information Sheet FS72), London, Parkinson's Disease Society.
27 B. McCall (2002) *Skin, Scalp and Sweating* (Parkinson's Disease Society Information Sheet FS40), London, Parkinson's Disease Society.
28 C. Cosgrove (2004) *Foot-care* (Parkinson's Disease Society Information Sheet FS51), London, Parkinson's Disease Society.
29 Interview with Geraldine Peacock (Winter 2003–4) *The Parkinson*, Parkinson's Disease Society, pp. 12–13.
30 B. Ramaswamy, R. Webber (2003) *Keeping Moving* (Booklet B74), London, Parkinson's Disease Society.
31 Interview with B. Thompson (Summer 2002) *The Parkinson*, Parkinson's Disease Society, pp. 12–13.
32 Interview with C. Johnson Wahl (Winter 2004) *The Parkinson*, Parkinson's Disease Society, pp. 14–15.
33 A. Iliff, N. Tingey (Summer 2000) 'The role of art therapy in Parkinson's', *The Parkinson*, Parkinson's Disease Society, pp. 14–15.
34 N. Tingey (Summer 2004) Catalyst: Art for Parkinson's, *Focus*, European Parkinson's Disease Association, 27, pp. 4–5.
35 Taken from B. McCall (2003) *International Travel* (Parkinson's Disease Society Information Sheet FS28), London, Parkinson's Disease Society.
36 From 'What is depression?', available from the Depression Alliance website (http://www.depressionalliance.org).
37 M. Jahanshahi, C. D. Marsden (2000) *Parkinson's Disease: a self-help guide*, New York, Demos Medical Publishing, p. 19.
38 S. Andersen (Summer 2004) *Focus*, European Parkinson's Disease Association, p. 2.
39 C. Stallibrass, C. Chalmers (2002) 'Randomized controlled trial of the Alexander technique for idiopathic Parkinson's disease', *Clinical Rehabilitation*, 16 pp. 705–18.
40 K. S. Schneider, T. Gold (1998) 'After the tears', *People*.
41 Taken from a presentation on Parkinson's disease given by Dr Doug

MacMahon at the British Geriatrics Society United in Care conference, held at the Royal College of Physicians, London, December 2004; the conference report can be read at <http://www.mepltd.co.uk> (accessed September 2005).

42   J. Meara and BK Bhowmick (2000) 'Parkinson's disease and parkinson-ism in the elderly', in J. Meara, W. C. Koller (eds) *Parkinson's and Parkinson's Disease in the Elderly*, Cambridge, Cambridge University Press, p. 22.

Index

134

new developments 116; research 57; tiredness 17; for tremors 6

emotions: attitudes 90–1; coping with diagnosis 29–31, 83–4; counselling 89; younger people 102
encephalitis 6–7
entacapone 50, 116
environmental factors: neuroprotection 12; neurotoxins 11
Ernst, Prof. Edzard 93
essential tremor condition 5–6
European Parkinson's Disease Association (EPDA) 30, 90, 92
Excel 2000 77
exercise and sport 76–8

family and friends: carers 112–15; relationships 84–6
finances 70–1
flunarizine 55
Foundation September: *Parkinson's Disease Self-Care Manual* 87
Fox, Michael J.: Foundation 29, 96–7; *Lucky Man* 83, 102–3
freezing 16

gamma knife surgery 61
genetic factors 10–12
Grimshaw, Rosalind 79
The Guardian 69, 72

hallucinations 53–4, 89
handwriting 18–19
head injuries 13
Health is Between Your Ears: Living with a Chronic Disease (EPDA) 90
health professionals 34–8, 42; nurse specialists 29, 34
herbal medicines 56
hobbies and travel 77–82
Holidays and Respite Care Guide (PDS) 81, 115
Huntington's disease 100

Jahanshahi, Marjan: *Parkinson's Disease: A Self-Help Guide* (with Marsden) 89
jobs 71–2, 95; carers 114; young-onset 104

Keeping Moving (Ramaswamy and Webber) 76

lesioning surgery 61, 64
levodopa 7, 45–6, 48, 116; younger people 100
Lewy bodies 4; genetic factors 11
lisuride 47
Lucky Man (Fox) 83, 102–3

magnetic resonance imaging (MRI) 26–7, 64
Marsden, C. David: *Parkinson's Disease: A Self-Help Guide* (with Jahanshahi) 89
mental abilities 89
methyldopa 56
metoclopramide 54
monoamine oxidase B inhibitors 51–2
multiple system atrophy (MSA) 6
muscular system: cramps 16; dystonia 16 *see also* rigidity; slowness; tremors

National Electronic Library for Health 93
National Health Service (NHS): carers 114; day hospitals and rehabilitation centres 38; Expert Patients programme 91–2; Patient Advice and Liaison Services 38–9
neuroimaging 26–8
neuroleptics 55–6
neuronal transplants 61
The New Role of the Patient (EPDA) 90

occupational therapy 35
orphenadrine 53

Parkinson, Dr James: *An Essay on the Shaking Palsy* 1
parkinsonism: age factors 107, 108; definition and types of 2–8; drug-induced 56, 107
Parkinson's Association of Ireland 102
Parkinson's disease: causes and factors 9–13; common symptoms 14–20; diagnosis of 24–32, 100; first description 1; information and resources 90–3; new developments